D1440874

Current Clinical Strategies

History and Physical Examination in Medicine

Second Edition

Paul D. Chan, M.D.
Peter J. Winkle, M.D.

Current Clinical Strategies Publishing
www.CCSPublishing.com

Current Clinical Strategies on the Internet

Visit the CCS Publishing internet site, where CCS online journals and books can be ordered.

http://www.CCSPublishing.com

Journal of Primary Care Medicine Online
Journal of Medicine Online
Journal of Pediatric Medicine Online
Journal of Surgery Online
Journal of Family Medicine Online
Journal of Emergency Medicine and Acute Primary Care
Journal of Psychiatry Online
Journal of AIDS/HIV

Digital Book and Updates

The digital book and updates of this text can be downloaded via the internet at the CCS Publishing URL: http://www.CCSPublishing.com

Current Clinical Strategies Publishing Inc
27071 Cabot Road, Suite 126
Laguna Hills, California 92653-7012
Phone: 800-331-8227
Fax: 800-965-9420
E-mail: info@CCSPublishing.com

Printed in USA   ISBN 1881528-17-0

Contents

Medical Documentation

History and Physical Examination

History

Identifying Data: Patient's name; age, race, sex. Name of informant (patient, relative).

Chief Compliant: Reason given by patient for seeking medical care.

History of Present Illness (HPI): Describe the course of the patient's illness, including when it began, character of the symptoms, location where the symptoms began; aggravating or alleviating factors; pertinent positives and negatives, and other related diseases. Describe past illnesses or surgeries, and past diagnostic testing.

Past Medical History (PMH): Past diseases, surgeries, hospitalizations; medical problems; history of diabetes, hypertension, peptic ulcer disease, asthma, myocardial infarction, cancer, tuberculosis. In children include birth history, prenatal history, immunizations, and type of feedings.

Medications:

Allergies: Penicillin?

Family History: Medical problems in family, including problems similar to patient's disorder. Asthma, myocardial infraction, heart failure, cancer, tuberculosis, diabetes.

Social History: Alcohol, smoking, drug usage. Marital status, employment situation. Level of education.

Review of Systems (ROS):

General: Weight gain or loss, loss of appetite, fever, chills, fatigue, night sweats.

Skin: Rashes, bruising, skin discolorations.

Head: Headaches, dizziness, masses, seizures, head trauma.

Eyes: Visual changes, visual field deficits.

Ears: Tinnitus, vertigo, hearing loss.

Nose: Nose bleeds, discharge, sinus diseases.

Mouth and Throat: Dental disease, hoarseness, throat pain.

Respiratory: Cough, shortness of breath, sputum (color), tuberculosis.

Cardiovascular: Chest pain, orthopnea, paroxysmal nocturnal dyspnea; dyspnea on exertion, claudication, edema, valvular disease.

Gastrointestinal: Dysphagia, abdominal pain, nausea, vomiting, hematemesis, diarrhea, constipation, melena (black tarry stools), hematochezia (bright red blood per rectum).

Genitourinary: Dysuria, frequency, hesitancy, hematuria, discharge.

Gynecological: Gravida/para, abortions, last menstrual period (frequency, duration), age of menarche, menopause; dysmenorrhea, contraception, vaginal bleeding, breast masses.

Endocrine: Polyuria, polydipsia, polyphagia, skin or hair changes, cold or heat intolerance.

Musculoskeletal: Joint pain or swelling, arthritis, myalgias.

Skin and Lymphatics: Easy bruising, lymphadenopathy.

Neuropsychiatric: Weakness, seizures, memory changes, depression.

Physical Examination

Vital Signs: Temperature, heart rate, respirations, blood pressure.

Skin: Rashes, scars, moles, capillary refill (in seconds).

Lymph Nodes: Cervical, supraclavicular, axillary, inguinal nodes; size, tenderness.

Head: Bruising, masses. In pediatric patients check fontanels.

Eyes: Pupils equal round and react to light and accommodation (PERRLA); extra ocular movements intact (EOMI), visual fields and acuity. Funduscope (papilledema, arteriovenous nicking, hemorrhages, exudates); scleral icterus, ptosis (drooping lid).

Ears: Acuity, tympanic membranes (dull, shiny, intact, injected, bulging).

Mouth and Throat: Mucus membrane color and moisture; oral lesions, dentition, pharynx, tonsils.

Neck: Jugular venous distention (JVD) at a 45 degree incline, thyromegaly, lymphadenopathy, masses, bruits, abdominojugular reflux.

Chest: Equal expansion, tactile fremitus, percussion, auscultation, rhonchi, crackles, rubs, breath sounds, egophony, whispered pectoriloquy.

Heart: Point of maximal impulse (PMI), thrills (palpable turbulence); regular rate and rhythm (RRR), first and second heart sounds (S1 and S2); gallops (S3, S4), murmurs (grade 1-6), pulses (graded 0-2+).

Breast: Dimpling, tenderness, lumps, nipple discharge.

Abdomen: Contour (flat, scaphoid, obese, distended); scars, bowel sounds, bruits, tenderness, masses, liver span by percussion; hepatomegaly, splenomegaly; guarding, rebound, percussion note (tympanic), costovertebral angle tenderness (CVAT), suprapubic tenderness.

Genitourinary: Skin lesions, inguinal masses, hernias, scrotum, testicles, varicoceles.

Pelvic Exam: Vaginal mucosa, cervical discharge, uterine size, masses, adnexa, ovaries.

Extremities: Joint swelling, range of motion, edema (grade 1-4+); cyanosis, clubbing, edema (CCE); pulses (radial, ulnar, femoral, popliteal, posterior tibial, dorsalis pedis; simultaneous palpation of radial and femoral pulses); cyanosis, varicosities.

Rectal Exam: Sphincter tone, masses, fissures; test for occult blood, prostate (nodules, tenderness, size).

Neurological: Mental status and affect; gait, strength (graded 0-5); touch sensation, pressure, pain, position and vibration; deep tendon reflexes (biceps, triceps, patellar, ankle; graded 0-4+); Romberg's test (ability of patient to stand erect with arms outstretched and eyes closed).

Cranial Nerve Examination:

  I: Smell

  II: Vision and visual fields

  III, IV, VI: Pupil responses to light, extraocular eye movements, ptosis

  V: Facial sensation, ability to open jaw against resistance, corneal reflex.

  VII: Close eyes tightly, smile, show teeth

  VIII: Hears watch tic; Weber test (lateralization of sound when tuning fork is placed on top of head); Rinne test (air conduction last longer than bone conduction when tuning fork is placed on mastoid process)

  IX, X: Palette moves in midline when patient says "ah," speech

  XI: Shoulder shrug and turns head against resistance

  XII: Stick out tongue in midline

Labs: Electrolytes (sodium, potassium, bicarbonate, chloride, BUN, creatinine), CBC (hemoglobin, hematocrit, WBC count, platelets, differential); x-rays, ECG, urine analysis (UA), liver function test (LFT's).

Assessment (Impression): Assign a number to each problem and discuss separately. Discuss differential diagnosis and give reasons to support the working diagnosis; give reasons for excluding other diagnoses.

Plan: Describe therapeutic plan for each numbered problem including testing, laboratory studies, medications, antibiotics.

Problem-Oriented Daily Progress Note

Problem List: List each problem separately (heart failure, pneumonia, hypokalemia). State hospital day number, post-operative day number, and antibiotic day number.

Subjective: Describe how the patient feels in the patient's own words; and give observations about the patient.

Objective: Vital signs, physical exam for each system, laboratory data.

Assessment: Evaluate each numbered problem, and discuss the progress of each problem.

Plan: For each problem, discuss any additional orders, changes in drug regimen or plans for discharge or transfer.

Discharge Summary

Patient's Name and Medical Record Number:
Date of Admission:
Date of Discharge:
Admitting Diagnosis:
Discharge Diagnosis:
Attending or Ward Team Responsible for Patient:
Surgical Procedures, Diagnostic Tests, Invasive Procedures:
Brief History, Pertinent Physical Examination and Laboratory Data: Describe the course of the patient's disease up until the patient came to the hospital including physical exam and laboratory data.

Hospital Course: Describe the course of the patient's illness while in the hospital, including evaluation, treatment, medications, outcome of treatment.

Discharged Condition: Describe improvement or deterioration in patient's condition, and describe his present status.

Disposition: Describe the situation to which the patient will be discharged (home, nursing home), and indicate who will take care of patient.

Discharged Medications: List medications and instructions for patient on taking the medications.

Discharged Instructions and Follow-up Care: Date of return for follow-up care at clinic; diet, exercise.

Problem List: List all active and past problems.

Copies: Send copies to attending, clinic, consultants.

Cardiovascular Disorders

Chest Pain and Myocardial Infarction

History: Duration of chest pain in hours. Location, radiation (to arm, jaw, back), character (squeezing, sharp, dull), intensity, rate of onset (gradual or sudden); relationship of pain to activity (at rest, during exercise); relief by nitroglycerine; increase in frequency or severity of baseline anginal pattern. Improvement or worsening of pain; occurrence during sleep.

Associated Symptoms: Diaphoresis, nausea, vomiting, dyspnea, orthopnea, edema, palpitations, dysphagia, cough, sputum, paresthesias, syncope.

Aggravating and Relieving Factors: Effect of inspiration or position on pain; effect of eating, NSAIDS, alcohol, exertion, stress.

Cardiac Testing: Past stress testing, angiograms, nuclear scans, ECG's.

Risk Factors for Coronary Heart Disease: Family history of coronary artery disease before age 55, diabetes, hypertension, smoking, hypercholesterolemia.

PMH: History of diabetes, claudication, stroke. Exercise tolerance; history of peptic ulcer disease, melena; menopausal status. Prior history of myocardial infarction, coronary bypass grafting or angioplasty.

Social History: Cocaine usage, elicit drugs, smoking, alcohol.

Medications: Aspirin, beta-blockers, estrogen replacement, nicotine replacement therapy.

Physical Exam

General: Visible pain, apprehension, distress, pallor.

Vitals P (tachycardia), BP in both arms, R (tachypnea), T.

Skin: Cold extremities (peripheral vascular disease), xanthomas (hypercholesterolemia).

HEENT: Fundi, "silver wire" arteries, arteriolar narrowing, A-V nicking, hypertensive retinopathy; carotid pulse amplitude, duration; carotid bruits; jugular venous distention.

Chest: Crackles, percussion note, friction rub.

Heart: Decreased intensity of first heart sound (S1) (LV dysfunction); third heart sound (S3) (heart failure, dilation), S4 gallop (more audible in the left lateral position; decreased LV compliance due to ischemia); mitral insufficiency murmur (papillary muscle dysfunction), cardiac rub (pericarditis).

Abdomen: Epigastric tenderness (peptic ulcer), hepatomegaly, ascites, pulsatile mass (aortic aneurysm).

Rectal: Occult blood.

Extremities: Edema, femoral bruits, unequal or diminished pulses (aortic dissection); calf pain, swelling (thrombosis).

Labs

Electrocardiographic Findings in Acute Myocardial Infarction

    A. ST segment elevations in two contiguous leads with ST depressions in reciprocal leads are strong predictors of MI and the need for primary angioplasty or thrombolysis. The earliest signs of transmural injury are hyperacute T waves. Q waves occur later.

CXR: Cardiomegaly, pulmonary edema (CHF).

LDH, Mg, CBC, electrolytes. CPK with isoenzymes, troponin I or troponin T, myoglobin, and LDH. Echocardiography.

Differential Diagnosis of Chest Pain

    A. **Acute Pericarditis.** Characterized by pleuritic-type chest pain and diffuse ST segment elevation.

    B. **Aortic Dissection.** "Tearing" chest pain with uncontrolled hypertension, widened mediastinum and increased aortic prominence on chest x-ray.

    C. **Esophageal Rupture** usually occurs after vomiting; x-ray may reveal air in mediastinum or a left side hydrothorax.

    D. **Acute Cholecystitis** is characterized by right subcostal abdominal pain with anorexia, nausea, vomiting, and fever.

    E. **Acute Peptic Ulcer Disease.** Epigastric pain with melena or hematemesis and anemia.

Dyspnea

History: Rate of onset of shortness of breath (gradual, sudden), orthopnea (shortness of breath when supine), paroxysmal nocturnal dyspnea (PND), chest pain, palpitations. Affect of physical exertion; history of myocardial infarction, syncope. Past episodes; aggravating or relieving factors (noncompliance with medications, salt overindulgence). Edema, weight gain, lightheadedness, cough, sputum, fever, nausea, fatigue, anxiety; leg pain (DVT).

Past Medical History: Bronchitis, emphysema, heart failure, hypertension, occupational exposures, coronary artery disease, HIV risk factors, history of asthma.

Medications: Bronchodilators, cardiac medications (noncompliance), drug allergies.

Past Treatment or Testing: Cardiac testing, x-rays, ECG's, spirometry.

Physical Exam

General: Respiratory distress. Fluid input and output balance.

Vitals: BP (supine and upright), P (tachycardia), T, R (tachypnea).

HEENT: Jugular venous distention at 45 degrees, tracheal deviation (pneumothorax).

Chest: Stridor (foreign body), retractions, breath sounds, wheezing, crackles (rales), rhonchi; dullness to percussion (pleural effusion), barrel chest; unilateral hyperresonance (pneumothorax).

Heart: Lateral displacement of point of maximal impulse, irregular, irregular rhythm (atrial fibrillation); S3 gallop (LV dilation), S4 (myocardial infarction), holosystolic apex murmur (mitral regurgitation); faint heart sounds (pericardial effusion).

Abdomen: Abdominojugular reflux (pressing on abdomen produces increased jugular vein distention), hepatomegaly, liver tenderness.

Extremities: Edema, pulses, cyanosis, clubbing, jaundice. Calf tenderness or swelling (DVT).

Labs: ABG, cardiac enzymes; CXR (cardiomegaly, hyperinflation with flattened diaphragms, infiltrates, effusions, pulmonary edema), ventilation/perfusion scan.

Electrocardiogram

A. ST segment depression or elevation, Q waves, or new left bundle-branch block.

B. ST elevations in two contiguous leads, with ST depressions in reciprocal leads, are strong predictors of MI.

Differential Diagnosis: Heart failure, myocardial infarction, upper airway obstruction, pneumonia, pulmonary embolism, chronic obstructive pulmonary disease, asthma, pneumothorax, foreign body aspiration, hyperventilation, malignancy, anemia.

Edema

History: Duration of edema; localized or generalized; associated pain, redness. History of heart failure, liver, or renal disease; weight changes, shortness of breath, malnutrition, chronic diarrhea (protein losing enteropathy), thyroid disease, prolonged sitting or immobility, estrogens, allergies, alcoholism. Exacerbation by menses, position.

Past Treating and Testing: Cardiac testing, chest x-rays. History of deep vein thrombosis, venous insufficiency, varicose veins. Recent fluid input and output balance.

Meds: Cardiac drugs, furosemide, diuretics, calcium channel blockers.

Physical Exam

Vitals: BP (orthostatic), P, T, R.

HEENT: Jugular venous distention at 45°; carotid pulse, amplitude, duration.

Chest: Breath sounds, crackles, wheeze, dullness to percussion.

Heart: Displacement of point of maximal impulse, atrial fibrillation (irregular, irregular); S3 gallop (LV dilation), rubs.

Abdomen: Abdominojugular reflux, ascites, hepatomegaly, splenomegaly, distention, fluid wave, shifting dullness.

Extremities: Pitting or non-pitting edema, varicose veins, redness, warmth; mottled, brown discoloration of ankle skin (venous insufficiency); leg circumference, tenderness, Homan's sign (dorsiflexion elicits pain; thrombosis); pulses, cyanosis, clubbing.

Labs: Electrolytes, liver function tests, CBC, chest x-ray, ECG, cardiac enzymes, Doppler studies of lower extremities.

Differential Diagnosis

Unilateral Edema: Venous obstruction (DVT, thrombophlebitis); lymphatic obstruction (neoplasm - pelvic, lymphoma).

Generalized Edema: Renal disease (acute glomerulonephritis, nephrotic syndrome, renal failure), cardiac disease (CHF), liver disease (cirrhosis, obstruction of hepatic venous outflow), vascular disease (AV fistula, obstruction of inferior or superior vena cava).

Endocrine: Mineralocorticoid excess, hypoalbuminemia (protein losing enteropathy, malnutrition).

Miscellaneous: Chronic anemia, angioedema (hereditary/acquired), iatrogenic edema.

Congestive Heart Failure

History: Duration of dyspnea; gradual or sudden onset; paroxysmal nocturnal dyspnea (PND), orthopnea; number of pillows needed under back when supine to prevent dyspnea; dyspnea on exertion (DOE); edema of lower extremities. Exercise tolerance (past and present). Weight gain. Patient's subjective opinion of severity of dyspnea compared with past episodes and the degree of physical impairment should be determined.

Associated Symptoms: Fatigue, chest pain, pleuritic pain, cough, fever, chills, sputum, nausea, diaphoresis, palpitations, nocturia, syncope, prior viral illness.

Past Medical History: Past episodes of heart failure; hypertension, excess salt or fluid intake; noncompliance with diuretics, digoxin, antihypertensives; alcoholism, drug use, diabetes, coronary artery disease, myocardial infarction, heart murmur, arrhythmias. Thyroid disease, anemia, pulmonary disease.

Past Testing: Echocardiograms for ejection fraction, cardiac testing, nuclear scans, angiograms, ECG's.

Risk Factors: Smoking, diabetes, family history of coronary artery disease or heart failure, hypercholesterolemia, hypertension.

Precipitating Factors: Infections, noncompliance with low salt diet; excessive fluid intake; anemia, hyperthyroidism, pulmonary embolism, nonsteroidal anti-inflammatory drugs, renal insufficiency; adverse drug reactions (beta blockers, calcium blockers, antiarrhythmics).

Treatment in Emergency Room: IV Lasix given, volume diuresed. Recent fluid input and output balance.

Physical Exam

General: Respiratory distress, anxiety, diaphoresis.

Vitals: BP (hypotension or hypertension), P (tachycardia), T, R (tachypnea).

HEENT: Jugular venous distention at 45 degree incline (measure vertical distance from the sternal angle to top of column of blood); hepatojugular reflux (pressing on abdomen causes jugular venous distention); carotid pulse, amplitude, duration, bruits.

Chest: Breath sounds, crackles, rhonchi; dullness to percussion (pleural effusion).

Heart: Lateral displacement of point of maximal impulse; irregular, irregular rhythm (atrial fibrillation); S3 gallop (LV dilation).

Abdomen: Ascites, hepatomegaly, liver tenderness.

Extremities: Edema, pulses, jaundice, muscle wasting.

Labs: CXR: Cardiomegaly, perihilar congestion; vascular cephalization (increased density of upper lobe vasculature); Kerley B lines (horizontal streaks in lower lobes), pleural effusions.

ECG: Left ventricular hypertrophy, ectopic beats, atrial fibrillation.

Electrolytes, BUN, creatinine, sodium; CBC; serial cardiac enzymes, CPK, MB, LDH. Echocardiogram.

Differential Diagnosis of Conditions That Mimic or Provoke Heart Failure:

- A. Coronary artery disease and myocardial infarction
- B. Hypertension
- C. Aortic or mitral valve disease
- D. Cardiomyopathies: Hypertrophic, idiopathic dilated, postpartum, genetic, toxic, nutritional, metabolic
- E. Myocarditis: Infectious, toxic, immune
- F. Pericardial constriction
- G. Tachyarrhythmias or bradyarrhythmias
- H. Pulmonary embolism
- I. Pulmonary disease
- J. High output states: Anemia, hyperthyroidism, A-V fistulas, Paget's disease, fibrous dysplasia, multiple myeloma
- K. Renal failure, nephrotic syndrome

Factors that Precipitate Heart Failure

- A. Increase Demand: Anemia, fever, infection, excess dietary salt, renal failure, liver failure, thyrotoxicosis, AV fistula, pregnancy. Arrhythmias, cardiac ischemia/infarction, pulmonary emboli, alcohol abuse, uncontrolled hypertension.
- B. Medication Related: Antiarrhythmics (disopyramide), negative inotropic agents (beta-blockers, calcium blockers), steroids, NSAID's, noncompliance with diuretics, excessive intravenous fluids

New York Heart Association Classification of Heart Failure

Class I: Symptomatic only with strenuous activity.

Class II: Symptomatic with usual level of activity.

Class III: Symptomatic with minimal activity, but asymptomatic at rest.

Class IV: Symptomatic at rest.

Palpitations and Atrial Fibrillation

History: Palpitations (rapid or irregular heart beat), fatigue, dizziness, nausea, dyspnea, edema; duration of atrial fibrillation. Results of previous ECG's.

Associated Symptoms: Chest pain, pleuritic pain, syncope, weakness, fatigue, diaphoresis, symptoms of hyperthyroidism.

Cardiac History: Hypertension, coronary disease, rheumatic heart disease, cardiomyopathies, arrhythmias, exercise intolerance.

Underlying Conditions: Pneumonia, diabetes, noncompliance with cardiac medications, pericarditis, hyperthyroidism, pulmonary embolism, pneumothorax, theophylline, myocardial infarction, electrolyte abnormalities, COPD, mitral valve stenosis, hypokalemia; diet pills, decongestants, alcohol, caffeine, cocaine.

Physical Exam

Vitals: BP (hypotension), P (irregular, irregular tachycardia).

HEENT: Retinal hemorrhages, jugular venous distention, carotid bruits; thyromegaly (hyperthyroidism).

Chest: Crackles (rales).

Heart: Irregular, irregular rhythm; dyskinetic apical pulse, displaced point of maximal impulse (cardiomegaly), S4, murmur (rheumatic fever); pericardial rub (pericarditis).

Rectal: Occult blood.

Extremities: Peripheral pulses with irregular timing and amplitude. Edema, cyanosis, ecchymoses, petechia (emboli). Femoral artery bruits (atherosclerosis).

Neuro: Motor weakness (hemiparesis), CN 2-12, sensory; dysphasia, dysarthria (stroke); tremor (hyperthyroidism).

Labs: Sodium, potassium, BUN, creatinine; magnesium; drug levels; CBC; serial cardiac enzymes; CPK, LDH, TSH, free T4. CXR.

ECG: Irregular R-R intervals with no P waves. Irregular baseline with rapid fibrillary waves (more than 320 per minute). The usual ventricular response rate is 130-180 per minute.

Echocardiogram for atrial chamber size.

Differential Diagnosis of Atrial Fibrillation

Lone Atrial Fibrillation: No underlying disease state.

Cardiac Causes: Hypertensive heart disease with left ventricular hypertrophy, heart failure, mitral valve stenosis or regurgitation, pericarditis, hypertrophic cardiomyopathy, coronary artery disease, myocardial infarction, aortic stenosis, infiltrative diseases (amyloidosis, cardiac tumors).

Noncardiac Causes: Hypoglycemia, theophylline intoxication, acute pulmonary disease (pneumonia, asthma, chronic obstructive pulmonary disease, pulmonary embolus), heavy alcohol intake or alcohol withdrawal, hyperthyroidism, severe acute stress or systemic illness, electrolyte abnormalities. Stimulant abuse, excess tobacco, caffeine, over-the-counter cold remedies, illicit drugs.

Hypertension

History: Degree of blood pressure elevation; patient's baseline BP from records; paroxysmal or sustained hypertension; baseline BUN and creatinine. Age of onset of hypertension.

Associated Symptoms: Chest or back pain (aortic dissection), dyspnea, orthopnea, dizziness, blurred vision (hypertensive retinopathy); nausea, vomiting, headache (pheochromocytoma); lethargy, confusion (encephalopathy).

Paroxysms of tremor, palpitations, diaphoresis; edema, thyroid disease, angina; flank pain, dysuria, polyuria, urinary infections. Alcohol withdrawal, noncompliance with antihypertensives (clonidine or beta-blocker withdrawal), excessive salt, alcohol.

Medications: Over-the-counter cold remedies, beta agonists, diet pills, ocular medications (sympathomimetics), bronchodilators, cocaine, amphetamines, nonsteroidal anti-inflammatory agents, oral contraceptives, adrenal steroids, MAO-inhibitors.

Risk Factors for Coronary Artery Disease: Family history of coronary artery disease before age 55, diabetes, hypertension, smoking, hypercholesterolemia.

Past Testing: Urinalysis, ECG, creatinine.

Physical Exam
General: Delirium, confusion, agitation (hypertensive encephalopathy).
Vitals: Supine and upright blood pressure (with correct size cuff; 2 readings); BP in all extremities.
HEENT: Hypertensive retinopathy, hemorrhages, exudates, "cotton wool" spots, A-V nicking; papilledema; thyromegaly (hyperthyroidism). Jugular venous distention, carotid bruits.

Chest: Crackles (rales, pulmonary edema), wheeze, intercostal bruits (aortic coarctation).

Heart: Rhythm; laterally displaced, sustained, forceful, apical impulse with patient in left lateral position (ventricular hypertrophy); narrowly split S2 with increased aortic component; systolic ejection murmurs (aorta outflow turbulence).

Abdomen: Renal bruits (systolic and diastolic bruit just below costal margin, renal artery stenosis); abdominal aortic enlargement or pulsations (aortic aneurysm); renal masses, enlarged kidney (polycystic renal disease); costovertebral angle tenderness. Truncal obesity (Cushing's syndrome).

Skin: Striae, skin atrophy (Cushing's syndrome), uremic frost (chronic renal failure); hirsutism (adrenal hyperplasia); plethora (pheochromocytoma).

Extremities: Asymmetric or delayed femoral to radial pulses; simultaneous palpation of femoral and brachial pulses (coarctation of aortic); femoral bruits, edema (peripheral vascular disease); tremor (pheochromocytoma, hyperthyroidism).

Neuro: Mental status, rapid return phase of deep tendon reflexes (hyperthyroidism), localized weakness (stroke), cranial nerve palsies, visual acuity.

Labs: Potassium, BUN, creatinine, glucose, calcium, uric acid, CBC. UA with microscopic analysis (RBC casts, hematuria, proteinuria). 24 hour urine for metanephrines, plasma catecholamines (pheochromocytoma), plasma renin activity.

12 lead electrocardiography may document evidence of ischemic heart disease, rhythm and conduction disturbances, or left ventricular hypertrophy.

CXR: Cardiomegaly, indentation of aorta (coarctation), rib notching.

Findings Suggesting Secondary Hypertension

    A. **Primary Aldosteronism.** Initial serum potassium <3.5 mEq/L while not taking medication.

    B. **Aortic Coarctation.** Femoral pulse delayed later than radial pulse or posterior systolic bruits below ribs.

    C. **Pheochromocytoma.** Orthostatic hypotension, tachycardia, tremor, pallor.

    D. **Renovascular Stenosis.** Paraumbilical abdominal bruits.

    E. **Polycystic Kidneys.** Flank or abdominal mass.

    F. **Pyelonephritis.** Persistent urinary tract infections, costovertebral angle tenderness.

    G. **Renal Parenchymal Disease.** Increased serum creatinine $\geq$1.5 mg/dL, proteinuria.

Screening Tests for Secondary Hypertension	
Renovascular Hypertension	Captopril Test: Plasma renin level before and 1 hr after captopril 25 mg PO. A greater than 150% increase in renin is positive Captopril Renography: renal scan before and after 25 mg PO Intravenous pyelography MRI angiography Arteriography (DSA)
Hyperaldosteronism	Serum Potassium 24 hr urine potassium Plasma renin activity CT scan of adrenals
Pheochromocytoma	24 hr urine metanephrine Plasma catecholamine level CT scan Nuclear MIBG scan
Cushing's Syndrome	Plasma ACTH Dexamethasone suppression test
Hyperparathyroidism	Serum calcium Serum parathyroid hormone

Differential Diagnosis of Hypertension

A. **Primary (essential) Hypertension (90%)**
B. **Secondary Hypertension:** Renovascular hypertension, pheochromocytoma, cocaine use; withdrawal from alpha2 stimulants, clonidine or beta blockers, or alcohol; noncompliance with antihypertensive medications.

Pericarditis

History: Sharp pleuritic chest pain; onset, intensity, radiation. Exacerbated by supine position, coughing or deep inspiration; relieved by leaning forward; referred to trapezius ridge; fever, chills, palpitations.

History of recent upper respiratory infection, autoimmune disease; prior episodes; tuberculosis exposure; intravenous drug abuse, dyspnea; myalgias, arthralgias, rashes, fatigue, anorexia, weight loss, kidney disease.

Medications: Hydralazine, procainamide, isoniazid, penicillin.

Physical Exam

Vitals: BP, P (tachycardia); pulsus paradoxus (drop in systolic BP >10 mmHg with inspiration).

HEENT: Cornea, sclera, iris lesions, oral ulcers (lupus); jugular venous distention (cardiac tamponade).

Skin: Malar rash (butterfly rash), discoid rash (lupus).

Chest: Crackles (rales), rhonchi.

Heart: Rhythm; friction rub on end-expiration while sitting forward; cardiac rub with 1-3 components at lower left sternal border; distant heart sounds (pericardial effusion).

Rectal: Occult blood.

Extremities: Arthralgias, arthritis.

Labs: ECG: diffuse, downwardly, concave, ST segment elevation in all 3 standard limb leads and several precordial leads; upright T waves, PR segment depression, low QRS voltage.

CXR: large cardiac silhouette; "water bottle sign"; pericardial calcifications.

Echocardiogram.

Increased WBC; UA, urine protein, RBC's; CPK, MB, LDH, blood culture, increased ESR.

Differential Diagnosis: Idiopathic, infectious (viral, bacterial, mycoplasmal, mycobacterial), Lyme disease, uremia, neoplasm, connective tissue disease, lupus, rheumatic fever, polymyositis, myxedema, sarcoidosis, post myocardial infarction (Dressler's syndrome), drugs (penicillin, isoniazid, procainamide, hydralazine).

Syncope

History: Time and description of the episode. Duration of unconsciousness, rate of onset; activity before and after event. Body position, arm position (reaching), neck position (turning to side); mental status before and after event. Precipitants (fear, tension, hunger, pain), cough, micturition, swallowing, defecation, exertion, Valsalva, hyperventilation, tight shirt collar. Seizure activity (tonic/clonic activity). Chest pain, palpitations.

Prodromal Symptoms: Nausea, diaphoresis, pallor, lightheadedness, dimming vision (vasovagal syncope).

Post-syncopal disorientation, confusion, vertigo, flushing; dyspnea, urinary of fecal incontinence, tongue biting. Rate of return to alertness (delayed or spontaneous), weakness.

Past Medical History: History of prior syncope, stroke, transient ischemic attacks, seizures, cardiac disease, arrhythmias, diabetes, anxiety attacks, exercise. Past Testing: 24 hour Holter, cardiac testing, ECG, EEG.

Medications Associated with Syncope	
Antihypertensives\Anti-angina agents	Antiarrhythmics
Adrenergic antagonists	Digoxin
Calcium channel blockers	Quinidine
Diuretics	Insulin
Nitrates	Drugs of abuse
Vasodilators	Alcohol
Antidepressants	Cocaine
Tricyclic antidepressants	Marijuana
Phenothiazines	

Physical Exam

General: Level of alertness.

Vitals: T, R, postural vitals (supine and after standing 2-5 minutes), P. Blood pressure in all extremities; simultaneous comparison of pulse intensity in extremities (aortic dissection).

HEENT: Cranial bruising (trauma). Pupil size and reactivity, extraocular movements; tongue or buccal lacerations (seizure); flat jugular veins (volume depletion); carotid or vertebral bruits.

Skin: Turgor, capillary refill, pallor.

Chest: Crackles, rhonchi (aspiration).

Heart: Irregular rhythm (atrial fibrillation); systolic murmurs (aortic stenosis), cardiac rub.

Abdomen: Bruits, tenderness pulsatile mass.

Genitourinary/Rectal: Occult blood, urinary or fecal incontinence (seizure).

Extremities: Palpate extremities for trauma.

Neuro: Cranial nerves 2-12, strength, gait, sensory, memory, tendon reflexes, mental status; nystagmus. Turn patient's head side to side, up and down; have patient reach above head, bend down and pick up object.

Labs: ECG: Arrhythmias, blocks. CXR, electrolytes, glucose, Mg, BUN, creatinine, CBC; EEG, 24-hour Holter monitor.

Differential Diagnosis of Syncope	
Non-cardiovascular	**Cardiovascular**

Metabolic
    Hyperventilation
    Hypoglycemia
    Hypoxia
Neurologic
    Cerebrovascular insufficiency
    Normal pressure hydrocephalus
    Seizure
    Subclavian steal syndrome
    Increased intracranial pressure
Psychiatric
    Hysteria
    Major depression
	Reflex (heart structurally normal)
	    Vasovagal
	    Situational
	    Cough
	    Defecation
	    Micturition
	    Postprandial
	    Sneeze
	    Swallow
	    Carotid sinus syncope
	Orthostatic hypotension
	Drug-induced
	Cardiac
	    Obstructive
	    Aortic dissection
	    Aortic stenosis
	    Cardiac tamponade
	    Hypertrophic cardiomyopathy
	    Left ventricular dysfunction
	    Myocardial infarction
	    Myxoma
	    Pulmonary embolism
	    Pulmonary hypertension
	    Pulmonary stenosis
	    Arrhythmias
	        Bradyarrhythmias
	            Sick sinus syndrome
	            Pacemaker failure
	        Supraventricular and ventricular
	            tachyarrhythmias

24 Syncope

Pulmonary Disorders

Hemoptysis

History: Quantify the amount of blood, acuteness of onset, color (bright red, dark), character (coffee grounds, clots), dyspnea, chest pain (left or right side), fever, chills, past bronchoscopies, exposure to tuberculosis; hematuria, weight loss, anorexia, malaise, hoarseness.

Farm exposure, homelessness, residence in a nursing home or prison, immigration from foreign country. Smoking, leg pain or swelling (pulmonary embolism), bronchitis, pneumonia, COPD, heart failure, anticoagulants, aspirin, NSAID's, HIV risk factors (pulmonary Kaposi's sarcoma), aspiration of food or foreign body.

Family history of bleeding disorders.

Prior chest X-rays, tuberculin testing (PPD).

Physical Exam

General: Dyspnea, respiratory distress.

Vitals: T, R (tachypnea), P (tachycardia), BP (hypotension); assess hemodynamic status.

HEENT: Nasal or oropharyngeal lesions; telangiectasias on buccal mucosa (Rendu-Osler-Weber disease); ulcerations of nasal septum (Wegener's granulomatosis), jugular venous distention, gingival disease (aspiration).

Lymph Nodes: Cervical, scalene or supraclavicular adenopathy (Virchow's nodes, intrathoracic malignancy).

Chest: Stridor, tenderness of chest wall; rhonchi, apical crackles (tuberculosis); localized wheezing (foreign body, malignancy), basilar crackles (pulmonary edema), pleural friction rub, breast masses (metastasis).

Heart: Mitral stenosis murmur (diastolic rumble), right ventricular gallop; accentuated, loud, second heart sound (pulmonary embolism).

Abdomen: Masses; liver nodules (metastases), tenderness.

Extremities: Petechiae, ecchymoses (coagulopathy); cyanosis, tenderness, calf swelling (pulmonary embolism); clubbing (pulmonary disease or cancer), edema, bone pain (metastasis).

Rectal: Occult blood.

Skin: Purple plaques (Kaposi's sarcoma); rashes (paraneoplastic syndromes).

Labs: Sputum Gram stain, cytology, acid fast bacteria stain; CBC, platelets,

ABG; pH of expectorated blood (alkaline=pulmonary; acidic=GI); UA (hematuria); PT/PTT, bleeding time, creatinine, fungal culture; anti-glomerular basement membrane antibody, antinuclear antibody; PPD, coccidioidomycosis serology.

EKG, chest x-ray, CT scan, bronchoscopy, arteriography, radionuclide scanning.

Differential Diagnosis

Infection: Bronchitis, pneumonia, lung abscess, tuberculosis, fungal infection, bronchiectasis, broncholithiasis.

Neoplasms: Bronchogenic carcinoma, metastatic cancer, Kaposi's sarcoma.

Vascular: Pulmonary embolism, mitral stenosis, pulmonary edema.

Miscellaneous: Trauma, foreign body, bleeding diathesis (anticoagulation), epistaxis, oropharyngeal bleeding, vasculitis, Goodpasture's syndrome, lupus, hemosiderosis, Wegener's granulomatosis, pulmonary aneurysm rupture.

Wheezing and Asthma

History: Onset, duration, and progression of wheezing; patient's subjective opinion of severity of attack; dyspnea, cough, fever, chills, purulent sputum; frequency of exacerbations and hospitalizations; history of steroid dependency, intubation, home oxygen or nebulizer use; peak flow rate

Exposure to allergens (foods, pollen, animals, drugs); activities or seasons that provoke symptoms; exacerbation by exercise, aspirin, beta- blockers, new medications, recent upper respiratory infection; chest pain, edema, foreign body aspiration.

Treatment given in emergency room and response.

Past Pulmonary History: Course of previous episodes of asthma; COPD, pneumonia, smoking. Baseline arterial blood gas results; past pulmonary function testing.

Family History: Family history of asthma, allergies, hay-fever, atopic dermatitis. Home dust control measures.

Physical Exam

General: Dyspnea, respiratory distress, diaphoresis, somnolence.

Vitals: T, R (tachypnea >28/min), P (tachycardia), BP (widened pulse pressure, hypotension), pulsus paradoxus (inspiratory drop in systolic blood pressure; >10 mmHg = severe attack).

HEENT: Nasal flaring, pharyngeal erythema. Cyanosis, jugular venous distention, grunting.

Chest: Prolonged expiratory wheeze, rhonchi, decreased intensity of breath sounds (emphysema);sternocleidomastoids muscle contractions, barrel chest, increased anteroposterior diameter (hyperinflation), intracostal and supraclavicular retractions.

Heart: Decreased cardiac dullness to percussion (hyperinflation); distant heart sounds, third heart sound gallop (S3, cor pulmonale), increased intensity of pulmonic component of second heart sound (pulmonary hypertension).

Abdomen: Retractions, tenderness.

Extremities: Cyanosis, edema, clubbing.

Skin: Atopic dermatitis, urticaria.

Neuro: Decreased mental status, confusion.

Labs: CXR: hyperinflation, bullae, flattening of diaphragms; small, elongated heart.

ABG: respiratory alkalosis, hypoxia.

Sputum gram stain; CBC, electrolytes, theophylline level.

ECG: sinus tachycardia, right axis deviation, right ventricular hypertrophy. Pulmonary function tests, peak flow rate.

Differential Diagnosis: Asthma, bronchitis, COPD, pneumonia, acute left ventricular heart failure, anaphylaxis, upper airway obstruction, carcinoid, endobronchial tumors.

Chronic Obstructive Pulmonary Disease

History: Duration of wheezing, dyspnea, cough, fever, chills; increased sputum production; sputum quantity, consistency, color; smoking (pack-years); chest trauma, noncompliance with medications. Patient's subjective opinion of severity of attack. Baseline blood gases.

Associated Symptoms: Chest pain, pleurisy. Adverse drug reactions (NSAIDS, beta blockers, sedatives), allergic reaction.

Past History: Frequency of exacerbations, home oxygen use, steroid dependency, history of intubations, nebulizer use; pneumonia, past pulmonary function tests.. Diabetes, heart failure, family history of emphysema, alcohol abuse.

Treatment given in Emergency Room.

Physical Exam

General: Diaphoresis, respiratory distress; speech interrupted by breaths, cachexia,

Vitals: T, R (tachypnea), P (tachycardia), BP.

HEENT: Pursed-lip breathing, jugular venous distention. Mucous membrane or perioral cyanosis.

Chest: Barrel chest, retractions, accessory muscle use (sternocleidomastoids), supraclavicular retractions, prolonged expiratory wheezing, rhonchi. Decreased air movement in the chest, hyperinflation.

Heart: Right ventricular heave, distant heart sounds, S3 gallop (cor pulmonale).

Extremities: Cyanosis, edema, clubbing.

Neuro: Decreased mental status, somnolence, confusion.

Labs: CXR: Diaphragmatic flattening, bullae, hyperaeration.

ABG: Respiratory alkalosis (early), acidosis (late), hypoxia. Sputum gram stain, culture, CBC, electrolytes.

ECG: Sinus tachycardia, right axis deviation, right ventricular hypertrophy, PVC's.

Differential Diagnosis: COPD, emphysema, chronic bronchitis, asthma, pneumonia, heart failure, alpha-1-antitrypsin deficiency, cystic fibrosis, kyphoscoliosis, obstructive sleep apnea.

Pulmonary Embolism

History: Sudden onset of pleuritic chest pain and dyspnea. Unilateral leg pain, swelling; fever, cough, hemoptysis, diaphoresis, syncope. History of deep vein thrombosis.

Virchow's Triad: Immobility, trauma, hypercoagulability; malignancy (pancreas, lung, genitourinary, stomach, breast, pelvic, bone); estrogens (oral contraceptives), history of heart failure, surgery, obesity, pregnancy.

Physical Exam

General: Dyspnea, apprehension, diaphoresis.

Vitals: T (fever), R (tachypnea, >16/min), P (tachycardia >100/min), BP (hypotension).

HEENT: Jugular venous distention, prominent jugular A-waves.

Chest: Crackles (rales); tenderness or splinting of chest wall, pleural friction rub; breast mass (malignancy).

Heart: Right ventricular gallop; accentuated, loud, pulmonic component of second heart sound (S2); S3 or S4 gallop; murmur.

Extremities: Cyanosis, edema calf redness, tenderness, Homan's Sign (pain with dorsiflexion of foot), warmth; swelling, increased calf circumference (>2 cm difference), dilated superficial veins, elevated skin temperature.

Rectal: Occult blood.

Genitourinary: Testicular or pelvic masses.

Neuro: Altered mental status.

Frequency of Symptoms and Signs in Pulmonary Embolism			
Symptoms	**%**	**Signs**	**%**
Dyspnea	84	Tachypnea (>16/min)	92
Pleuritic chest pain	74	Rales	58
Apprehension	59	Accentuated S2	53
Cough	53	Tachycardia	44
Hemoptysis	30	Fever (>37.8°C)	43
Sweating	27	Diaphoresis	36
Non-pleuritic chest pain	14	S3 or S4 gallop	34
Syncope	13	Thrombophlebitis	32

Labs: ABG: Hypoxemia, hypocapnia, respiratory alkalosis.

Lung Scan: Ventilation/perfusion mismatch. Duplex imaging and impedance plethysmography of lower extremities.

Pulmonary angiogram: Arterial filling defects.

CXR: Elevated hemidiaphragm, wedge shaped infiltrate; localized oligemia; effusion, segmental atelectasis.

ECG: Sinus tachycardia, nonspecific ST-T wave changes, QRS changes (acute right shift, S_1Q_3 pattern); right heart strain pattern (P-pulmonale, right bundle branch block, right axis deviation).

Differential Diagnosis: Heart failure, myocardial infarction, pneumonia, pulmonary edema, chronic obstructive pulmonary disease, asthma, aspiration of foreign body or gastric contents, hyperventilation.

30 Pulmonary Embolism

Infectious Diseases

Fever and Sepsis

History: Degree of fever; time of onset, pattern of fever; shaking chills (rigors), cough, sputum, sore throat, headache, neck stiffness, dysuria, frequency; night sweats; vaginal discharge, back pain; myalgias, nausea, vomiting, diarrhea, malaise, anorexia.

Chest or abdominal pain, ear, bone or joint pain; recent antipyretic use. Cirrhosis, diabetes, valvular disease, recent surgery; AIDS risk factors, prosthetic implants; central IV lines.

Exposure to tuberculosis or hepatitis; travel history, animal exposure; recent dental GI procedures. Ill contacts; IV or Foley catheter; antibiotic or alcohol use. Recent WBC differential, allergies.

Physical Exam

General: Lethargy, toxic appearance, altered level of consciousness.

Vitals: Temperature (fever curve), R (tachypnea or hypoventilation), P (tachycardia), BP (hypotension).

HEENT: Papilledema; dental infection, tympanic membrane inflammation, sinus tenderness; pharyngeal erythema, lymphadenopathy, neck rigidity.

Breast: Tenderness, masses.

Chest: Rhonchi, crackles, dullness to percussion (pneumonia).

Heart: Murmurs (endocarditis).

Abdomen: Masses, liver tenderness, hepatomegaly, splenomegaly; Murphy's Sign (right upper quadrant tenderness and arrest of respiration secondary to pain, cholecystitis); shifting dullness, ascites. Costovertebral angle or suprapubic tenderness.

Extremities: Cellulitis, infected decubitus ulcers or wounds; IV catheter tenderness (phlebitis), calf tenderness, Homan's sign; joint or bone tenderness (septic arthritis). Osler's nodes, Janeway's lesions (peripheral lesions of endocarditis). Poor muscle tone

Rectal: Prostate tenderness; rectal flocculence, fissures, ulcers.

Pelvic/Genitourinary: Foley catheter; pelvic exam, cervical discharge, cervical motion tenderness; adnexal or uterine tenderness, masses; genital herpes lesions.

Skin: Pallor, cool extremities, delayed capillary refill; rash, purpura, petechia (septic emboli, meningococcemia), ecthyma gangrenosum (purpuric necrotic plaque of Pseudomonas infection). Pustules, cellulitis, furuncles, abscesses, cysts.

Labs: CBC, blood C&S x 2, glucose, BUN, creatinine, UA, urine Gram stain, C&S; lumbar puncture; blood, urine, skin lesion cultures, bilirubin, transaminases, alkaline phosphatase; tuberculin skin test, Gram Strain of buffy coat

CXR; abdomen X-ray; gallium, indium scans.

Laboratory Tests for Serious Infections	
Complete blood count, including leukocyte differential and platelet count	Cultures with antibiotic sensitivities
	Blood
Electrolytes	Urine
Arterial blood gases	Endometrium (if endometritis suspected)
Blood urea nitrogen and creatinine	Amniotic fluid (if chorioamnionitis suspected)
Urinalysis	
INR, partial thromboplastin time, fibrinogen	Wound
Serum lactate	Other sites (eg, sputum, drains)
	Chest X-ray
	Adjunctive imaging studies (eg, computed tomography, magnetic resonance imaging, abdominal X-ray)

Differential Diagnosis

Infectious Causes: Abscesses, mycobacterial infections (tuberculosis), cystitis, pyelonephritis, endocarditis, wound infection, diverticulitis, cholangitis, osteomyelitis, IV catheter phlebitis, sinusitis, otitis media, upper respiratory infection, pharyngitis, pelvic infection, cellulitis, hepatitis, infected decubitus ulcer, furuncle, peritonitis, abdominal abscess, perirectal abscess, AIDS, mastitis; viral, parasite infections.

Malignancies: Lymphomas, leukemia, solid tumors, carcinomas.

Connective Tissue Diseases: Lupus, rheumatic fever, rheumatoid arthritis, temporal arteritis, sarcoidosis, polymyalgia rheumatica.

Other Causes of Fever: Atelectasis, drug fever, pulmonary emboli, pericarditis, pancreatitis, factitious fever, alcohol withdrawal. Deep vein thrombosis, myocardial infarction, gout, porphyria, thyroid storm.

Medications Associated with Fever: Barbiturates, hydralazine, isoniazid, methyldopa, nitrofurantoin, penicillins, phenytoin, procainamide, sulfonamides.

Cough and Pneumonia

History: Duration of cough, chills, rigors, fever; rate of onset of symptoms. Sputum color, quantity, consistency, blood; living situation (nursing home, homelessness). Recent antibiotic use.

Associated Symptoms: Pleuritic chest pain, dyspnea, sore throat, rhinorrhea, headache, stiff neck, ear pain; nausea, vomiting, diarrhea, myalgias, arthralgias.

Past Pulmonary History: Previous pneumonia, intravenous drug abuse, AIDS risk factors. Diabetes, heart failure, COPD, asthma, immunosuppression, alcoholism, steroids; ill contacts, aspiration, smoking, travel history, exposure to tuberculosis. Pneumococcal vaccination, tuberculin testing.

Physical Exam

General: Respiratory distress, dehydration.

Vitals: T (fever), R (tachypnea), P (tachycardia), BP.

HEENT: Tympanic membranes, pharyngeal erythema, lymphadenopathy, neck rigidity.

Chest: Dullness to percussion, tactile fremitus (increased vocal conduction); rhonchi; end-inspiratory crackles; bronchial breath sounds with decreased intensity; whispered pectoriloquy (increased transmission of sound), egophony (E to A changes).

Extremities: Cyanosis, clubbing.

Neuro: Gag reflex, mental status.

Labs: CBC, electrolytes, BUN, creatinine, glucose; UA, ECG. ABG.

CXR: segmental consolidation, air bronchograms, atelectasis, effusion.

Sputum Gram stain: >25 WBC per low-power field, bacteria.

Differential Diagnosis: Pneumonia, heart failure, asthma, bronchitis, viral infection, pulmonary embolism, malignancy.

Etiologic Agents of Community Acquired Pneumonia

Age 5-40 (without underlying lung disease): Viral, mycoplasma pneumoniae, chlamydia pneumoniae (TWAR), streptococcus pneumoniae, legionella.

>40 (no underlying lung disease): Streptococcus pneumonia, group A streptococcus, H. influenza.

>40 (with underlying disease): Klebsiella pneumonia, Enterobacteriaceae, Legionella, Staphylococcus aureus, Chlamydia pneumoniae.

Aspiration Pneumonia: Streptococcus pneumoniae, bacteroides sp., anaerobes, Klebsiella, Enterobacter.

Pneumocystis Carinii Pneumonia and AIDS

History: Progressive exertional dyspnea and inability to perform usual activities (climbing stairs). Fever, chills, insidious onset of symptoms; CD4 lymphocyte count and HIV-RNA titer (viral load); duration of HIV positivity; prior episodes of PCP or opportunistic infection.

Dry nonproductive cough (or productive of white, frothy sputum), night sweats. Prophylactic trimethoprim/sulfamethoxazole treatment; antiviral therapy. Baseline and admission arterial blood gas.

Associated Symptoms: Headache, stiff neck, lethargy, fatigue, weakness, malaise, weight loss, diarrhea, visual changes. Oral lesions, odynophagia (painful swallowing), skin lesions.

Past Infectious Disease History: History of herpes simplex, toxoplasmosis, tuberculosis, hepatitis, mycobacterium avium complex, syphilis. Prior pneumococcal immunization. Mode of acquisition of HIV infection; sexual, substance use history (intravenous drugs), blood transfusion.

Medications: Antivirals, prescribed and alternative medications.

Physical Exam

General: Cachexia, respiratory distress, cyanosis

Vitals: T (fever), R (tachypnea), P (tachycardia), BP (hypotension).

HEENT: Herpetic lesions; oropharyngeal thrush, hairy leukoplakia; oral Kaposi's sarcoma (purple-brown macules); retinitis, hemorrhages, perivascular white spots, cotton wool spots (CMV retinitis); visual acuity and visual field deficits (toxoplasmosis.)

Neck rigidity, lymphadenopathy.

Chest: Dullness, decreased breath sounds at bases; crackles.

Heart: Murmurs (IV drug users).

Abdomen: Right upper quadrant tenderness, hepatosplenomegaly.

Pelvic/Rectal: Candidiasis, anal herpetic lesions, ulcers, condyloma.

Dermatologic Stigmata of AIDS: Rashes, Kaposi's sarcoma (multiple purple nodules or plaques), seborrheic dermatitis, zoster, herpes, molluscum contagiosum; oral thrush.

Lymph Node Examination: Enlarged nodes.

Neuro: Confusion, disorientation (AIDS dementia complex, meningitis, encephalitis), motor, sensory, cranial nerves, visual field defects (toxoplasmosis).

Labs: CXR: Diffuse, interstitial infiltrates.

ABG: hypoxia, increased Aa gradient. CBC, sputum gram stain, Pneumocystis immunofluorescent stain; CD4 count, hepatitis surface antigen and antibody, electrolytes. Bronchoalveolar lavage, diffusion capacity for carbon monoxide, high resolution CT scan.

Differential Diagnosis: Pneumocystis carinii pneumonia, bacterial pneumonia, tuberculosis, Kaposi's sarcoma.

Meningitis

History: Duration and degree of fever, chills, rigors; headache, neck stiffness; cough, sputum; lethargy, irritability (high pitched cry in children), altered consciousness, nausea, vomiting, seizures. Skin rashes, dysuria, ill contacts, travel history.

History of pneumonia, bronchitis, otitis media, sinusitis, endocarditis. Diabetes, alcoholism, sickle cell disease, splenectomy malignancy, immunosuppression, AIDS, intravenous drug use, tuberculosis; recent upper respiratory infections, antibiotic use.

Physical Exam

General: Level of consciousness; obtundation, labored respirations.

Vitals: T (fever), P (tachycardia), R (tachypnea), BP (hypotension).

HEENT: Pupil size and reactivity, extraocular movements, papilledema. Full fontanelle in infants. Brudzinski's sign (neck flexion causes hip flexion); Kernig's sign (flexing hip and extending knee elicits resistance).

Chest: Rhonchi, crackles.

Heart: Murmurs.

Skin: Capillary refill, rashes, nail bed splinter hemorrhages, Janeway's lesions (Endocarditis), petechia, purpura (meningococcemia).

Neuro: Altered mental status, cranial nerve palsies, motor weakness, sensory deficits, Babinski's sign.

CT Scan: Increased intracranial pressure should be excluded.

Labs

  CSF Tube 1 - Gram stain, culture and sensitivity, bacterial antigen screen (1-2 mL).

  CSF Tube 2 - Glucose, protein (1-2 mL).

CSF Tube 3 - Cell count and differential (1-2 mL).

CBC, electrolytes, BUN, creatinine.

Differential Diagnosis: Meningitis, encephalitis, brain abscess, parameningeal infection, viral infection, tuberculosis. Cervical muscle strain, cervical disc disease, osteomyelitis, subarachnoid hemorrhage.

Etiology of Bacterial Meningitis

15 - 50 years: Streptococcus pneumoniae, N. meningitis, listeria.

>50 years or debilitated: Same as above plus - Hemophilus influenza, Pseudomonas, streptococci.

AIDS: Cryptococcus neoformans, Toxoplasma gondii, lymphoma, herpes encephalitis, coccidioides.

Cerebral Spinal Fluid Analysis

Disease	Color	Protein	Cells	Glucose
Normal CSF Fluid	Clear	<50 mg/100 mL	<5 lymphs/mm³	>40 mg/100 ml, 1/2-2/3 blood glucose drawn at same time
Bacterial meningitis early viral or tuberculous meningitis	Yellow opalescent	Elevated 50-1500	25-10000 WBC with predominate polys	low
Tuberculous, fungal, partially treated bacterial, syphilitic meningitis, meningeal metastases	Clear opalescent	Elevated usually <500	10-500 WBC with predominant lymphs	20-40, low
Viral meningitis, partially treated bacterial meningitis, and encephalitis, toxoplasmosis, parameningeal infection	Clear opalescent	Slightly elevated or normal	10-500 WBC with predominant lymphs	Normal to low

Pyelonephritis and Urinary Tract Infection

History: Dysuria, frequency (voiding repeatedly of small amounts), urgency; suprapubic discomfort or pain, hematuria, fever, chills, malaise (pyelonephritis); back pain, nausea, vomiting.

History of urinary infections, renal stones or colicky pain. Recent antibiotic use, prostate enlargement. Diaphragm use.

Risk factors: Diaphragm or spermicide use, sexual intercourse, elderly, anatomic abnormality, calculi, prostatic obstruction, urinary tract instrumentation. Urinary tract obstruction, catheterization.

Physical Exam

General: Signs of dehydration.

Vitals: T (fever), R, P, BP.

Abdomen: Suprapubic tenderness, costovertebral angle tenderness, masses.

Pelvic/Genitourinary: Urethral or vaginal discharge, cystocele.

Rectal: Prostatic hypertrophy or tenderness (prostatitis).

Labs: UA with micro. Urine Gram stain, urine C&S. CBC with differential, SMA7.

Pathogens: E coli, Klebsiella, Proteus, Pseudomonas, Enterobacter, Staphylococcus saprophyticus, enterococcus, group B strep, Chlamydia trachomatis.

Differential Diagnosis: Acute cystitis, pyelonephritis, vulvovaginitis, gonococcal or chlamydia urethritis, herpes, cervicitis, renal infarction, papillary necrosis, renal calculus, appendicitis, cholecystitis, pelvic inflammatory disease.

Endocarditis

History: Fever, chills, night sweats, fatigue, malaise, weight loss; pain in fingers or toes; pleuritic chest pain; skin lesions; history of heart murmur, rheumatic heart disease, heart failure, prosthetic valve.

Intravenous drug use, recent intravenous catheter, dental procedure; infection or instrumentation of urinary or gastrointestinal tract; colonic disease, decubitus ulcers, wound infection. History of stroke.

Physical Exam

Vitals: T (fever), P (tachycardia), BP (hypotension).

HEENT: Oral mucosal and conjunctival petechiae; Roth's spots (retinal hemorrhages with pale center; emboli).

Heart: New or worsening cardiac murmur.

Abdomen: Liver tenderness (abscess); splenomegaly, spinal tenderness (vertebral abscess).

Neuro: Focal neurological deficits (septic emboli).

Extremities: Splinter hemorrhages under nails; Osler's nodes (erythematous or purple tender nodules on pads of toes or fingers); Janeway lesions (erythematous nontender lesions on palms and soles, septic emboli), joint pain (septic arthritis).

Labs: WBC, UA (hematuria); blood cultures x 3, urine culture.

Echocardiogram: Vegetations, valvular insufficiency.

CXR: Cardiomegaly, valvular calcifications, multiple focal infiltrates.

Pathogens

Native Valve: Streptococcus viridans, streptococcus bovis, enterococci, staphylococcus aureus, streptococcus pneumonia, pseudomonas, group D streptococcus.

Prosthetic Valve: Staphylococcus aureus, Enterobacter sp., staphylococcus epidermidis.

40 Endocarditis

Gastrointestinal Disorders

Acute Abdomen and Abdominal Pain

History: Duration of pain, pattern of progression; location at onset and at present; diffuse or localized; location and character at onset and at present (burning, crampy, sharp, dull); constant or intermittent ("colicky"); radiation (to shoulder, back, groin); sudden or gradual onset.

Effect of eating, vomiting, defecation, flatus, urination, inspiration, movement, position. Timing and characteristics of last bowel movement. Similar episodes in past; relation to last menstrual period.

Associated Symptoms: Fever, chills, nausea, vomiting (bilious, feculent, undigested food, blood, coffee grounds); vomiting before or after onset of pain; jaundice, constipation, change in bowel habits or stool caliber, obstipation (inability to pass gas); chest pain, diarrhea, hematochezia (rectal bleeding); melena (black stools); dysuria, hematuria, anorexia, weight loss, dysphagia, odynophagia (painful swallowing); early satiety, trauma.

History of abdominal surgery (appendectomy, cholecystectomy, aortic graft), hernias, gallstones; coronary disease, kidney stones; alcoholism, cirrhosis, peptic ulcer, dyspepsia.

Past Treatment or Testing: Endoscopies, x-rays, upper GI series.

Aggravating or Relieving Factors: Fatty food intolerance, medications, aspirin, NSAID's, narcotics, anticholinergics, laxatives, antacids.

Physical Exam

General: Degree of distress, body positioning to relieve pain, nutritional status

Vitals: T (fever), P (tachycardia), BP (hypotension), R (tachypnea).

HEENT: Pale conjunctiva, scleral icterus, atherosclerotic retinopathy, "silver wire" arteries (ischemic colitis); flat neck veins (hypovolemia). Lymphadenopathy, Virchow node (supraclavicular mass).

Abdomen

Inspection: Scars, ecchymosis, visible peristalsis (small bowel obstruction), distension. Scaphoid, flat; exact point of maximal pain.

Auscultation: Absent bowel sounds (paralytic ileus or late obstruction), high-pitched rushes (obstruction), bruits (ischemic colitis).

Palpation: Begin palpation in quadrant diagonally opposite to point of maximal pain with patient's legs flexed and relaxed. Bimanual palpation of flank (renal disease or retrocecal appendix). Rebound tenderness;

hepatomegaly, splenomegaly, masses; hernias (incisional, inguinal, femoral). Pulsating masses; costovertebral angle tenderness. Bulging flanks, shifting dullness, fluid wave (ascites).

Specific Signs on Palpation

Murphy's sign (inspiratory arrest with right upper quadrant palpation, cholecystitis).

Charcot's sign (right upper quadrant pain, jaundice, fever; gallstones). Courvoisier's sign (palpable, nontender gallbladder with jaundice, pancreatic malignancy).

McBurney's point tenderness (located two thirds of the way between umbilicus and anterior superior iliac spine; appendicitis).

Iliopsoas sign (elevation of legs against examiner's hand causes pain, retrocecal appendicitis). Obturator sign (flexion of right thigh and external rotation of thigh causes pain in pelvic appendicitis).

Rovsing's sign (manual pressure and release at left lower quadrant colon causes referred pain at McBurney's point; appendicitis).

Cullen's sign (bluish periumbilical discoloration; peritoneal hemorrhage). Grey Turner's sign (flank ecchymoses; retroperitoneal hemorrhage).

Percussion: Loss of liver dullness (perforated viscus, free air in peritoneum); liver and spleen span by percussion.

Rectal Exam: Masses, tenderness, stool; gross or occult blood.

Genital/Pelvic Examination: Cervical discharge, adnexal tenderness, uterine size, masses, cervical motion tenderness.

Extremities: Femoral pulses, popliteal pulses (absent pulses indicate ischemic colitis) edema.

Skin: Jaundice, dependent purpura (mesenteric infarction), petechia (gonococcemia).

Stigmata of Liver Disease: Spider angiomata, periumbilical collateral veins (Caput medusae), gynecomastia, ascites, hepatosplenomegaly, testicular atrophy.

Labs: CBC, electrolytes, liver function tests, amylase, lipase, UA, pregnancy test. ECG.

Chest x-ray: Free air under diaphragm, infiltrate, effusion (pancreatitis).

X-rays of abdomen (acute abdomen series): Flank stripe, subdiaphragmatic free air, distended loops of bowel, sentinel loop, air fluid levels, thumb printing, mass effects, calcifications, fecaliths, portal vein gas, pneumatobilia.

Differential Diagnosis

Generalized Pain: Intestinal infarction, peritonitis, obstruction, diabetic ketoacidosis, sickle crisis, acute porphyria, penetrating posterior duodenal ulcer, psychogenic pain.

Right Upper Quadrant: Cholecystitis, cholangitis, hepatitis, gastritis, pancreatitis, hepatic metastases, gonococcal perihepatitis (Fitz-Hugh-Curtis syndrome), retrocecal appendicitis, pneumonia, peptic ulcer.

Epigastrium: Gastritis, peptic ulcer, gastroesophageal reflux disease, esophagitis, gastroenteritis, pancreatitis, perforated viscus, intestinal obstruction, ileus, myocardial infarction, aortic aneurysm.

Left Upper Quadrant: Peptic ulcer, gastritis, esophagitis, gastroesophageal reflux, pancreatitis, myocardial ischemia, pneumonia, splenic infarction, pulmonary embolus.

Left Lower Quadrant: Diverticulitis, intestinal obstruction, colitis, strangulated hernia, inflammatory bowel disease, gastroenteritis, pyelonephritis, nephrolithiasis, mesenteric lymphadenitis, mesenteric thrombosis, aortic aneurysm, volvulus, intussusception, sickle crisis, salpingitis, ovarian cyst, ectopic pregnancy, endometriosis, testicular torsion, psychogenic pain.

Right Lower Quadrant: Appendicitis, diverticulitis (redundant sigmoid) salpingitis, endometritis, endometriosis, intussusception, ectopic pregnancy, hemorrhage or rupture of ovarian cyst, renal calculus, regional enteritis.

Hypogastric/Pelvic: Cystitis, salpingitis, ectopic pregnancy, diverticulitis, strangulated hernia, endometriosis, appendicitis, ovarian cyst torsion; bladder distension, nephrolithiasis, prostatitis, malignancy.

Nausea and Vomiting

History: Character of emesis (color, food, bilious, feculent, hematemesis, coffee ground material, projectile); abdominal pain, effect of vomiting on pain; early satiety, fever, melena vertigo, tinnitus (labyrinthitis).

Clay colored stools, dark urine, jaundice (biliary obstruction); recent change in medications. Ingestion of spoiled food ; exposure to Ill contacts; dysphagia, odynophagia.

Possibility of pregnancy (last menstrual period, contraception, sexual history). Diabetes, cardiac disease, peptic ulcer, liver disease, CNS disease, headache.

Drugs Associated with Nausea: Digoxin, colchicine, theophylline, chemotherapy, anticholinergics, morphine, meperidine (Demerol), ergotamines, oral

contraceptives, progesterone, antiarrhythmics, erythromycin, antibiotics.
Past Testing: X-rays, upper GI series, endoscopy.

Physical Exam
Vitals: BP (orthostatic hypotension), P (tachycardia), R, T (fever).
Skin: Pallor, jaundice, spider angiomas.
HEENT: Nystagmus, papilledema; ketone odor on breath (apple odor, diabetic ketoacidosis); jugular venous distention.
Abdomen: Scars, bowel sounds, bruits, tenderness, rebound, rigidity, distention, hepatomegaly, ascites.
Extremities: Edema.
Rectal: Masses, occult blood.
Labs: CBC, electrolytes, UA, amylase, lipase, LFT's, pregnancy test, acute abdomen x-ray series.
Differential Diagnosis: Gastroenteritis, systemic infections, medications (contraceptives, antiarrhythmics, chemotherapy, antibiotics), pregnancy, appendicitis, cholecystitis, hepatitis, intestinal obstruction, peptic ulcer, gastroesophageal reflux, gastroparesis, ileus, pancreatitis, myocardial ischemia, tumors (esophageal, gastric) increased intracranial pressure, labyrinthitis, diabetic ketoacidosis, renal failure, toxins, bulimia, psychogenic.

Anorexia and Weight Loss

History: Time of onset, amount and rate of weight loss (sudden, gradual); change in appetite, nausea, vomiting, dysphagia, abdominal pain; exacerbation of pain with eating (intestinal angina); diarrhea, fever, chills, night sweats; dental problems; restricted access to food.
Polyuria, polydipsia; skin or hair changes; 24-hour diet recall; dyspepsia, jaundice, dysuria; cough, change in bowel habits; chronic medical illness.
Dietary restrictions (low salt, low fat); diminished taste, malignancy, AIDS risks factors; psychiatric disease, renal disease, alcoholism, drug abuse (cocaine, amphetamines).
Signs of depression: Weight change, change in appetite, loss of interest in usual activities, sleep abnormalities, decreased libido.

Physical Exam
General: Muscle wasting, cachexia.

Vitals: P (bradycardia), BP, R, T (hypothermia).

Skin: Pallor, jaundice, hair changes, skin laxity, cheilosis, dermatitis, glossitis (Pellagra).

HEENT: Dentition, oropharyngeal lesions, thyromegaly, glossitis, supraclavicular, temporal wasting, adenopathy (Virchow's node).

Chest: Rhonchi, barrel shaped chest.

Heart: Murmurs, displaced PMI.

Abdomen: Scars, decreased bowel sounds, tenderness, hepatomegaly splenomegaly. Periumbilical adenopathy, palpable masses.

Extremities: Edema, muscle wasting, lymphadenopathy.

Neuropathy: Decreased sensation, poor proprioception.

Rectal: Occult blood, masses.

Labs: CBC, electrolytes, protein, albumin, pre-albumin, transferrin, thyroid studies, LFT's, toxicology screen.

Differential Diagnosis: Inadequate dietary intake, peptic ulcer, depression, anorexia nervosa, dementia, hyper/hypothyroidism, cardiopulmonary disease," sedatives, psychotropics, digoxin, laxatives, thiazides, antibiotics, narcotics, diminished taste, diminished olfaction, poor dental hygiene (loose dentures), cholelithiasis, malignancy (gastric carcinoma), gastritis, hepatic or renal failure, systemic infection, alcohol abuse, AIDS, mesenteric ischemia.

Diarrhea

History: Rate of onset, duration, frequency, timing of the diarrheal episodes. Volume of stool output (number of stools per day), watery stools; fever. Cramping, abdominal cramps, bloating, flatulence, tenesmus (urge to defecate), anorexia, nausea, vomiting, ability to keep food or liquids down, bloating; lightheadedness, myalgias, arthralgias, headache, weight loss.

Stool Appearance: Buoyancy, blood or mucus, oily, foul odor.

Recent ingestion of spoiled poultry (salmonella), milk, seafood (shrimp, shellfish; Vibrio parahaemolyticus); common sources (restaurant), travel history.

Effect of fasting on diarrhea (osmotic diarrhea decreases with fasting, secretory diarrhea is unchanged with fasting), laxative abuse.

Ill contacts with diarrhea; inflammatory bowel disease, hyperthyroidism; family history of coeliac disease.

Sexual exposures, immunosuppressive agents, AIDS risk factors, coronary artery disease, peripheral vascular disease (ischemic colitis).

Exacerbation by stress, daytime only diarrhea with mucous stools (irritable bowel syndrome).

Drugs and Substances Associated with Diarrhea: Laxatives, magnesium-containing antacids, sulfa drugs, antibiotics (erythromycin, clindamycin), cholinergic agents, colchicine, milk (lactase deficiency), candy, gum (sorbitol).

Physical Exam

General: Signs of dehydration or malnutrition.

Vitals: BP (orthostatic hypotension), P (tachycardia), R, T (fever).

Skin: Skin turgor, delayed capillary refill, jaundice.

HEENT: Oral ulcers (inflammatory bowel or coeliac disease), dry mucous membranes, cheilosis (cracked lips, riboflavin deficiency); glossitis (B12, folate deficiency). Oropharyngeal candidiasis (AIDS).

Abdomen: Hyperactive bowel sounds, tenderness, rebound, hepatomegaly guarding, rigidity (peritoneal signs), distention; bruits (ischemic colitis).

Extremities: Arthritis, joint swelling (ulcerative colitis). Absent peripheral pulses or bruits (ischemic colitis).

Rectal: Perianal or rectal ulcers, sphincter tone, tenderness, masses, occult blood. Sphincter reflex.

Neuro: Mental status changes. Peripheral neuropathy (B6, B12 deficiency), decreased perianal sensation.

Labs: Electrolytes, Wright's stain for fecal leucocytes; cultures for enteric pathogens, ova and parasites x 3; clostridium difficile toxin. CBC with differential, calcium, albumen, flexible sigmoidoscopy.

Abdominal X-ray: Air fluid levels, dilation, pancreatic calcifications.

Differential Diagnosis

Acute Infectious Diarrhea: Infectious diarrhea (salmonella, shigella, E coli, Campylobacter, Staphylococcus aureus or Bacillus cereus, enteric virus (rotavirus, Norwalk virus), traveler's diarrhea, antibiotic-related diarrhea

Chronic Diarrhea:

Osmotic Diarrhea: Laxatives, lactulose, lactase deficiency (gastroenteritis, sprue), other disaccharidase deficiencies, ingestion of mannitol, nasogastric tube feeding, sorbitol.

Secretory Diarrhea: Bacterial enterotoxins, viral infection; AIDS associated disorders (mycobacterial, HIV), Zollinger-Ellison syndrome, vasoactive intestinal peptide tumor, carcinoid tumors, medullary thyroid carcinoma, colonic villus adenoma, terminal ileal disease with bile salt malabsorption.

Exudative Diarrhea: Bacterial infection, Clostridium difficile, parasites, Crohn's disease, ulcerative colitis, diverticulitis, chemotherapy, intestinal ischemia, radiation injury, diverticulitis with or without abscess.

Diarrhea Secondary to Altered Intestinal Motility: Diabetic gastroparesis, hyperthyroidism, laxatives, cholinergics, irritable bowel syndrome, "dumping syndrome," bacterial overgrowth (stasis related), constipation-related diarrhea.

Hematemesis and Upper Gastrointestinal Bleeding

History: Duration and frequency of hematemesis (bright red blood, coffee ground material), volume of blood, hematocrit. Forceful retching prior to hematemesis (Mallory-Weiss tear). Abdominal pain, melena, hematochezia (bright red blood per rectum); history of peptic ulcer, esophagitis, prior bleeding episodes. Ingestion of alcohol, aspirin, nonsteroidal anti-inflammatory drugs, steroids, anticoagulants; nose bleeds, syncope, lightheadedness, nausea.

Weight loss, malaise, fatigue, anorexia, early satiety, jaundice. History of liver or renal disease, hepatic encephalopathy, esophageal varices, aortic surgery.

Nasogastric aspirate quantity and character; transfusions given previously. Family history of liver, gastrointestinal disease or bleeding disorders.

Past Testing: x-ray studies, endoscopy.

Past Treatment: Endoscopic sclerotherapy, shunt surgery, treatment of prior episodes of GI bleeding.

Physical Exam

General: Pallor, diaphoresis, cold extremities, confusion.

Vitals: Supine and upright pulse and blood pressure (orthostatic hypotension); (resting tachycardia indicates a 10% blood volume loss; postural hypotension with increase pulse of 20 and decrease in systolic of 20 indicates a 20-30% blood loss); oliguria (<20 mL of urine per hour), T.

Skin: Delayed capillary refill, pallor, petechiae, ecchymosis. Stigmata of liver disease [jaundice, umbilical venous collaterals (caput medusae), spider angiomas, parotid gland hypertrophy]. Hemorrhagic telangiectasia (Osler-Weber-Rendu syndrome), abnormal pigmentation (Peutz-Jeghers syndrome); purple brown nodules (Kaposi's sarcoma).

HEENT: Scleral pallor, oral telangiectasia, flat neck veins.

Chest: Gynecomastia (cirrhosis), breast masses (metastatic disease).

Heart: Systolic ejection murmur.

Abdomen: Scars, tenderness, rebound, masses, splenomegaly, hepatic atrophy (cirrhosis), liver nodules. Ascites, dilated abdominal veins.

Extremities: Dupuytren's contracture (palmar contractures, cirrhosis), edema.

Neuro: Decreased mental status, confusion, poor memory, asterixis (flapping with wrists when hyperextended, hepatic encephalopathy).

Genitourinary/Rectal: Gross or occult blood, masses, testicular atrophy.

Labs: CBC, platelets, electrolytes, BUN (elevation suggests upper GI bleed), glucose, PT/PTT, ECG. Endoscopy, nuclear scan, angiography.

Differential Diagnosis of Upper Bleeding: Gastric or duodenal ulcer, esophageal varices, Mallory Weiss tear (gastroesophageal junction tear due to vomiting or retching), gastritis, esophagitis, swallowed blood (nose bleed, oral lesion), duodenitis, gastric cancer, vascular ectasias, coagulopathy, hypertrophic gastropathy (Menetrier's disease), aorto-enteric fistula.

Melena and Lower Gastrointestinal Bleeding

History: Duration, quantity, color of bleeding (gross blood, streaks on stool, melena), recent hematocrit. Change in bowel habits or stool caliber, abdominal pain, fever. Constipation, diarrhea, anorectal pain. Epistaxis, anorexia, weight loss, malaise, vomiting. Fecal mucus, tenesmus (straining during defecation), lightheadedness; history of diverticulosis, hemorrhoids, colitis, peptic ulcer, hematemesis, bleeding disease, coronary or renal disease, cirrhosis, alcoholism, easy bruising.

Anticoagulants, aspirin, NSAIDS.

Color of nasogastric aspirate.

Past Testing: Barium enema, colonoscopy, sigmoidoscopy, upper GI series.

Physical Exam

Vitals: BP, P (orthostatic hypotension), R, T (tachycardia), oliguria.

Skin: Cold, clammy skin; delayed capillary refill, pallor, jaundice. Stigmata of liver disease: Umbilical venous collaterals (Caput medusae), jaundice, spider angiomata, parotid gland hypertrophy, gynecomastia. Rashes, purpura; buccal mucosa discolorations or pigmentation (Henoch-Schönlein purpura or Peutz-Jeghers polyposis syndrome).

HEENT: Atherosclerotic retinal disease (ischemic colitis), "silver wire" arteries.

Heart: Systolic ejection murmurs; atrial fibrillation (mesenteric emboli).

Abdomen: Scars, bruits, masses, distention, rebound, tenderness, hernias, liver atrophy (cirrhosis), splenomegaly. Ascites, pulsatile masses (aortic aneurysm).

Genitourinary: Testicular atrophy.

Extremities: Cold, pale extremities.

Neuro: Decreased mental status, confusion, asterixis (flapping hand tremor; hepatic encephalopathy).

Rectal: Gross or occult blood, masses, hemorrhoids; fissures, polyps, ulcers.

Labs: CBC (anemia), liver function tests. Abdomen x-ray series (thumbprinting, air fluid levels).

Differential Diagnosis of Lower Gastrointestinal Bleeding: Hemorrhoids, fissures, diverticulosis, upper GI bleeding, rectal trauma, inflammatory bowel disease, infectious or ischemic colitis, bleeding polyps, carcinoma, angiodysplasias, intussusception, coagulopathies, Meckel's diverticulitis, epistaxis, small intestine tumor, endometriosis, aortoenteric fistula.

Cholecystitis

History: Duration of biliary colic (constant right upper quadrant pain, occurring 30-90 minutes after meals, lasting several hours). Radiation to right epigastrium, scapula or back; nausea, vomiting, anorexia, low grade fever; fatty food intolerance, dark urine, clay colored stools; bloating, jaundice, early satiety, flatulence, obesity.

Previous epigastric pain, gallstones, alcohol. History of fasting, rapid weight loss, hyperalimentation, estrogen, pregnancy, diabetes, sickle cell anemia, hereditary spherocytosis.

Prior Testing: Ultrasounds, HIDA scans, endoscopies.

Cholesterol Stones: Hereditary, pregnancy, exogenous steroids, diabetes, Crohn's disease, terminal ileal resection; rapid weight loss, hyperalimentation.

Pigment Stones: Asians with biliary parasites, hemolytic states (sickle cell anemia, hereditary spherocytosis), cirrhosis, biliary stasis.

Physical Exam

General: Obese, restless patient unable to find comfortable position.

Vitals: P (mild tachycardia), T (low-grade fever), R (shallow respirations), BP.

Skin: Jaundice

HEENT: Scleral icterus, sublingual jaundice.

Abdomen: Epigastric or right upper quadrant tenderness, Murphy's sign (tenderness and inspiratory arrest during palpation of RUQ); firm tender, sausage-like mass in RUQ (enlarged gallbladder); guarding, rigidity, rebound (peritoneal signs); Charcot's sign (intermittent right upper quadrant abdominal pain, jaundice, fever).

Labs: Ultrasound, HIDA (radionuclide) scan, WBC, hyperbilirubinemia, increased alkaline phosphatase, AST, amylase.

Plain Abdominal X-ray: increased gallbladder shadow, gallbladder calcifications; air in gallbladder wall (emphysematous cholecystitis), small bowel obstruction (gallstone ileus).

Differential Diagnosis: Calculus cholecystitis, acalculous cholecystitis, cholangitis, peptic ulcer, pancreatitis, appendicitis, gastroesophageal reflux disease, hepatitis, abscess, nephrolithiasis, pyelonephritis, hepatic metastases, gonococcal perihepatitis (Fitz-Hugh-Curtis syndrome), pleurisy, pneumonia, angina, pericarditis, herpes zoster.

Jaundice and Hepatitis

History: Dull right upper quadrant pain, anorexia, jaundice, nausea, vomiting, fever, dark urine, increased abdominal girth (ascites), pruritus, arthralgias, urticarial rash; somnolence (hepatic encephalopathy). Weight loss, melena, hematochezia, hematemesis. IV drug abuse, alcoholism, exposure to hepatitis or jaundiced persons, blood transfusion, oral-fecal exposure, day care centers, residential institutions; prior hepatitis immunization. Heart failure, sepsis.

Hepatotoxins: Acetaminophen, isoniazid, nitrofurantoin, methotrexate, sulfonamides, NSAIDS, phenytoin.

Family history of jaundice/liver disease.

Prior Testing: Hepatitis serologies, liver function tests, liver biopsy.

Physical Exam

Vitals: P, BP, R, T (fever).

Skin: Needle tracks, sclerotic veins (from intravenous injections), urticaria, bronze discoloration (hemochromatosis).

Stigmata of liver disease: Jaundice, umbilical venous collaterals (Caput medusae), spider angiomas, palmar erythema.

HEENT: Scleral icterus, sublingual jaundice, lymphadenopathy, Kayser-Fleischer rings (bronze corneal pigmentation, Wilson's disease).

Chest: Gynecomastia, Murphy's sign (cessation of inspiration with palpation of the right upper quadrant).

Abdomen: Scars, bowel sounds, right upper quadrant tenderness; liver span, hepatomegaly; liver margin texture (blunt, irregular, firm), splenomegaly (hepatitis) or hepatic atrophy (cirrhosis), ascites. Courvoisier's sign (palpable nontender gallbladder with jaundice; pancreatic or biliary malignancy).

Genitourinary: Testicular atrophy.

Extremities: Joint tenderness, palmar erythema, Dupuytren's contracture (fibrotic palmar ridge).

Neuro: Disorientation, confusion, asterixis (flapping when wrists are hyperextended, encephalopathy).

Rectal: Occult blood; hemorrhoids.

Labs: CBC with differential, LFT's, amylase, lipase, hepatitis serologies (hepatitis B surface antibody, hepatitis B surface antigen, hepatitis A IgM, hepatitis C antibody), antimitochrondrial antibody (primary biliary cirrhosis), ANA, ceruloplasmin, urine copper (Wilson's disease), alpha 1 antitrypsin deficiency, drug screen, serum iron, TIBC, ferritin (hemochromatosis), ultrasound, liver biopsy.

Differential Diagnosis of Jaundice

Extrahepatic: Biliary tract disease (gallstone, stricture, cancer), infections (parasites, HIV, CMV, microsporidia); acute pancreatitis, chronic pancreatitis with stricture, pancreatic cancer.

Intrahepatic: Viral hepatitis, medication-related, pregnancy (acute fatty liver), alcoholic hepatitis, cirrhosis, primary biliary cirrhosis, autoimmune hepatitis, Wilson's disease, right heart failure, total parenteral nutrition; hereditary deficiency (increased direct hyperbilirubinemia - Dubin Johnson syndrome, Rotor's syndrome; indirect - Gilbert's, Crigler-Niger), sclerosing cholangitis, Hodgkin disease, sarcoidosis, amyloidosis, tumor.

Cirrhosis

History: Jaundice, anorexia, nausea, fever; abdominal distension or pain, increased abdominal girth (ascites); vomiting, diarrhea, fatigue. Somnolence, confusion (encephalopathy); alcohol use. Viral hepatitis, blood transfusion, IV drug use.

Precipitating Factors of Encephalopathy: Gastrointestinal bleeding, high protein intake, constipation, azotemia, CNS depressants.

Physical Exam

General: Fetor hepaticas (odor of breath caused by mercaptans), muscle wasting.

Vitals: P, BP, T, R.

Skin: Jaundice, spider angiomas (stellate, erythematous arterioles), palmar erythema; bronze skin discoloration (hemochromatosis), purpura, loss of body hair.

HEENT: Kayser-Fleischer rings (bronze corneal pigmentation, Wilson's disease), jugular venous distention (fluid overload). Parotid enlargement, sclera icterus, gingival hemorrhage (thrombocytopenia).

Chest: Bibasilar crackles, gynecomastia.

Abdomen: Bulging flanks, tenderness, rebound (peritonitis); fluid wave, shifting dullness, "puddle sign" (examiner flicks over lower abdomen while auscultating for dullness). Courvoisier's sign (palpable nontender gallbladder with jaundice; pancreatic or Biliary malignancy); atrophic liver; liver margin texture (blunt, irregular, firm), splenomegaly. Umbilical or groin hernias (ascites).

Genitourinary: Edema of scrotum, testicular atrophy.

Extremities: Lower extremity edema.

Neuro: Confusion, asterixis (jerking movement of hand with wrist hyperextended; hepatic encephalopathy).

Rectal: Occult blood, hemorrhoids.

Stigmata of Liver Disease: Spider angiomas (stellate red arterioles), jaundice, bronze discoloration (hemochromatosis), dilated periumbilical collateral veins (Caput medusae), ecchymoses, umbilical eversion, venous hum and thrill at umbilicus (Cruveilhier-Baumgarten syndrome); palmar erythema, Dupuytren's contracture (fibrotic palmar ridge to ring finger). Lacrimal and parotid gland enlargement, testicular atrophy, gynecomastia, ascites, encephalopathy, edema.

Labs: CBC, electrolytes, LFT's, albumin, PT/PTT, liver function tests, bilirubin,

UA. Hepatitis serologies,, antimitochondrial, antibody (primary, biliary cirrhosis), ANA, anti-Smith antibody, ceruloplasmin, urine copper (Wilson's disease), alpha-1-antitrypsin, serum iron, TIBC, ferritin (hemochromatosis).

Abdominal x-ray: Hepatic angle sign (loss of lower margin of right, lateral, liver angle), separation or centralization of bowel loops, generalized abdominal haziness (ascites). Ultrasound, paracentesis.

Differential Diagnosis

Alcoholic liver disease, viral hepatitis (B, C, D), hemochromatosis, primary biliary cirrhosis, autoimmune hepatitis, inborn error of metabolism (Crigler Najjar syndrome; Wilson's disease, alpha 1 antitrypsin deficiency), heart failure, venous outflow obstruction (Budd-Chiari, portal vein thrombus).

Evaluation of Ascites Fluid

Etiology	Appearance	Protein	Serum/fluid albumen ratio	RBC	WBC	Other
Cirrhosis	Straw	<3 g/dL	>1.1	low	<250 cells/mm³	
Spontaneous Bacterial Peritonitis	Cloudy	<3	>1.1	low	>250 polys	Bacteria on gram stain and culture
Secondary Bacterial Peritonitis	Purulent	>3	<1.1	low	>10000	Bacteria on gram stain and culture
Neoplasm	Straw/bloody	>3	varies	high	>1000 lymphs	Malignant cells on cytology; triglycerides
Tuberculosis	Clear	>3	<1.1	low-high	>1000 lymphs	Acid fast bacilli
Heart Failure	Straw	>3	>1.1	low	<1000	
Pancreatitis	Turbid	>3	<1.1	varies	varies	Elevated amylase, lipase

Pancreatitis

History: Constant, dull, boring, mid-epigastric or left upper quadrant pain; radiation to the mid-back; exacerbated by supine position, relieved by sitting with knees drawn up; nausea, vomiting, low-grade fever, rigors, jaundice; anorexia, dyspnea; elevated amylase.

Precipitating Factors: Alcohol, gallstones, trauma, postoperative, retrograde cholangiopancreatography, trauma, hypertriglyceridemia, hypercalcemia, renal failure, viral (Coxsackie virus, mumps), or mycoplasma infection. Lupus, vasculitis, penetration of peptic ulcer, scorpion stings. Tumor, pancreatic divisum, sphincter of Oddi dysfunction.

Medications Associated with Pancreatitis: Sulfonamides, thiazides, dideoxyinosine (DDI), furosemide, tetracycline, estrogens, azathioprine, valproate, pentamidine.

Physical Exam

General: Signs of volume depletion, tachypnea.

Vitals: Low grade fever, tachycardia, hypotension.

Chest: Crackles, left lower lobe dullness (pleural effusion).

HEENT: Scleral icterus, Chvostek's sign (taping cheek results in facial spasm, hypocalcemia).

Skin: Jaundice, subcutaneous fat necrosis (erythematous skin nodules on legs and ankles). Palpable purpura (polyarteritis nodosum).

Abdomen: Epigastric tenderness, distension; rigidity, rebound, guarding, hypoactive bowel sounds; upper abdominal mass; Cullen's sign (periumbilical bluish discoloration from hemoperitoneum), Grey-Turner's sign (blue or greenish flank discoloration; retroperitoneal hemorrhage).

Extremities: Peripheral edema, anasarca.

Labs: Amylase, lipase, calcium, WBC, triglycerides, glucose, AST, LDL, UA.

Abdomen X-Rays: Ileus, pancreatic calcifications, obscure psoas margins, displaced or atonic stomach. Colon cutoff sign (spasm of splenic flexure with no distal colonic gas), diffuse ground-glass appearance of (ascites).

Chest x-ray: Left plural effusion.

Ultrasound: Gallstones, pancreatic edema or enlargement.

CT scan with oral contrast: Pancreatic phlegmon, pseudocyst, abscess.

Ranson's Criteria of Pancreatitis Severity.

Early criteria: Age >55; WBC >16,000; glucose >200; LDH >350 IU/L; AST >250.

During initial 48 hours: Hematocrit decrease >10%; BUN increase >5; arterial pO2 <60 mmHg; base deficit >4 mEq/L; calcium <8; estimated fluid sequestration >6 L.

Differential Diagnosis of Midepigastric Pain: Pancreatitis, peptic ulcer, cholecystitis, hepatitis, bowel obstruction, mesenteric ischemia, renal colic, aortic dissection, pneumonia, myocardial ischemia.

Factors Associated with Pancreatitis: Alcoholic pancreatitis, gallstone pancreatitis, penetrating peptic ulcer, trauma, medications, hyperlipidemia, hypercalcemia, infections (viral, ascaris), congenital disorders (pancreatic divisum, familial pancreatitis), pancreatic malignancy, toxins (methyl alcohol, scorpion bites), sphincter of Oddi dysfunction, endoscopic retrograde cholangiopancreatography, vasculitis.

Gastritis and Peptic Ulcer Disease

History: Recurring, dull, burning, epigastric pain; 1-3 hours after meals; relieved by or worsen by food; worse when supine or reclining; relieved by antacids; awakens patient at night or in early morning. May radiate to back; nausea, vomiting, weight loss, coffee ground hematemesis; melena. Smoking, alcohol, salicylates, nonsteroidal anti-inflammatory drugs.

History of previous examinations: Endoscopy upper GI series, surgery; history of previous ulcer disease and Helicobacter pylori (HP) therapy.

Physical Exam
General: Mild distress.
Vitals: P (tachycardia), BP (orthostatic hypotension), R, T.
Skin: Pallor, delayed capillary refill.
Abdomen: Mild to moderate epigastric tenderness; rebound, rigidity, guarding (perforated ulcer), bowel sounds.
Rectal: Occult blood.
Labs: CBC, electrolytes, BUN, amylase, lipase. Abdominal x-rays, endoscopy.
Differential Diagnosis: Pancreatitis, gastritis, gastroenteritis, perforating ulcer, intestinal obstruction, mesenteric adenitis, mesenteric thrombosis, aortic aneurysm, gastric dysmotility, gastroesophageal reflux disease, non-ulcer dyspepsia.

Mesenteric Ischemia and Infarction

History: Severe, poorly localized, mid-abdominal pain; pain is postprandial and may be relieved by nitroglycerine; bloody diarrhea, food aversion, weight loss, nausea, vomiting. Peripheral vascular disease, claudication, chest pain, coronary artery disease, atrial fibrillation, hypercholesterolemia, diabetes, CHF.

Physical Exam

General: Lethargy, mild to moderate distress.

Vitals: P, BP (orthostatic hypotension), P (tachycardia), R, T.

HEENT: Atherosclerotic retinopathy, "silver wire" arteries; carotid bruits (ischemic colitis).

Skin: Cold, clammy skin, pallor.

Abdomen: Initially hyperactive, then absent, bowel sounds; peritoneal signs (rebound, tenderness, rigidity, guarding), pulsatile masses (aortic aneurysm), abdominal bruit.

Extremities: Weak peripheral pulses, femoral bruits; asymmetric pulses (atherosclerotic disease).

Rectal: Occult or gross blood.

Labs: CBC, electrolytes, leukocytosis. Hemoconcentration, prerenal azotemia, serum lactic acid (metabolic acidosis).

Chest x-ray: Free air under diaphragm (perforated viscus). Abdominal x-ray: "thumb-printing" (edema of intestinal wall), portal vein gas. Bowel wall gas (colonic ischemia, nonocclusive); angiogram.

Differential Diagnosis. Peritonitis, acute appendicitis, acute cholecystitis, perforated viscus, peptic ulcer, gastroenteritis, pancreatitis, bowel obstruction, carcinoma, ruptured aortic aneurysm.

Intestinal Obstruction

History: Vomiting, obstipation, distention, crampy abdominal pain. Initially crampy or colicky pain with exacerbations at intervals of 5-10 minutes. Pain becomes diffuse with fever. Hernias, previous abdominal surgery, use of opiates, anticholinergics, antipsychotics, gallstones; colon cancer; history of constipation, vomiting.

Character of emesis (feculent, bloody). Pain localizes to periumbilical region in small bowel obstruction and localizes to lower abdomen in large bowel obstruction.

Physical Exam

General: Severe distress.

Vitals: BP (hypotension), P (tachycardia), R, T (fever).

Skin: Cold clammy skin, pallor.

Abdomen: Hernias (incisional, inguinal, femoral, umbilical), scars (intraabdominal adhesions).

Bowel Sounds: High pitch rushes (early) or absent bowel sounds (late).

Tenderness, rebound, rigidity, masses, distention, bruits.

Rectal: Gross blood, masses.

Labs: CBC, electrolytes; metabolic alkalosis due to vomiting, amylase.

Abdominal x-rays: dilated loops of small or large bowel, air-fluid levels, sentinel loop.

Causes of Small Bowel Obstruction: Adhesions (previous surgery), hernias, strictures from inflammatory processes; superior mesenteric artery syndrome, gallstone ileus. Ischemia, small bowel tumors, metastatic cancer.

Causes of Large Bowel Obstruction: Colon cancer, volvulus, diverticulitis, adynamic ileus, mesenteric ischemia, Ogilvie's syndrome (chronic pseudo-obstruction); narcotic ileus. Inflammatory bowel disease with stricture.

Differential Diagnosis: Myocardial infarction, gallstones, peptic ulcer, gastroenteritis, peritonitis, sickle crisis, cancer, pancreatitis, renal colic.

Gynecologic Disorders

Amenorrhea

History: Primary amenorrhea (absence of menses by age 16) or secondary amenorrhea (cessation of menses in a female with previously normal menstruation). Last menstrual period. Determine the menstrual pattern, timing of breast and pubic hair development, sexual activity (pregnancy).

Life style changes, dieting and excessive exercise, medications (contraceptives) or drugs (marijuana), stress.

Hot flushes and night sweats (hypoestrogenism), galactorrhea (prolactinoma).

History of dilation and curettage, postpartum infection (Asherman's syndrome) or hemorrhage (Sheehan's syndrome), obesity, weight gain or loss, headaches, visual disturbances, thyroid symptoms; symptoms of pregnancy (nausea, breast tenderness), phenothiazines, antidepressants. Prior pregnancies. Age of mother and sister(s) at menarche and menopause.

Assess diet, medications or drugs, and psychologic stress.

Previous radiation therapy, chemotherapy.

Physical Exam

General: Secondary sexual characteristics, body habitus, obesity, signs of hyperthyroidism or hypothyroidism.

HEENT: Acne, hirsutism, temporal balding, deepening of the voice, visual field defects, thyroid enlargement.

Chest: Galactorrhea, breast development, breast atrophy.

Abdomen: Abdominal striae (Cushing's syndrome).

Gyn: Pubic hair distribution. Inguinal or labial masses, clitoromegaly, vaginal obstruction, imperforate hymen, vaginal septum, vaginal atrophy, uterine enlargement, ovarian cysts or tumors.

Neuro: Focal motor deficits.

Labs: Pregnancy test, prolactin, TSH, free T_4. Progesterone-estrogen challenge testing.

Differential Diagnosis of Amenorrhea	
Pregnancy	**Outflow tract-related**
Hormonal contraception	Imperforate hymen
Hypothalamic-related	Transverse vaginal septum
Chronic or systemic illness	Agenesis of the vagina, cervix,
Stress	uterus
Athletics	Uterine synechiae
Eating disorder	**Androgen excess**
Obesity	Chronic anovulatory
Drugs	hyperandrogenism (PCO)
Tumor	Adrenal tumor
Pituitary-related	Adrenal hyperplasia (classic and
Hypopituitarism	nonclassic)
Tumor	Ovarian tumor
Infiltration	**Other endocrine causes**
Infarction	Thyroid disease
Ovarian-related	Cushing syndrome
Dysgenesis	
Agenesis	
Ovarian failure	
Resistant ovary	

Abnormal Uterine Bleeding

History: Last menstrual period, age of menarche; regularity, duration and frequency of menses; amount of bleeding, number of pads per day; passing of clots; postcoital or intermenstrual bleeding; pain, fever, chills, lightheadedness, sexual activity, possibility of pregnancy, birth control method. changes in hair or skin texture or distribution

Molimina symptoms (premenstrual breast tenderness, bloating, dysmenorrhea). Obstetrical history.

Thyroid, renal, or hepatic diseases, coagulopathies. Dental bleeding, stress, exercise, weight changes, genital trauma.

Family history of coagulopathies, endocrine disorders.

Physical Exam

General: Assess rate of bleeding. Obesity, hirsutism, petechiae, skin and hair changes.

Vitals: Assess hemodynamic stability, tachycardia, hypotension, orthostatic vitals, thyroid enlargement, galactorrhea.

Gyn: Cervical motion tenderness, adnexal tenderness, uterine size, cervical lesions. Cervical lesions should be biopsied.

Labs: CBC, platelets; serum pregnancy test; GC and chlamydia cultures, endometrial sampling. PT/PTT, type and screen.

Differential Diagnosis

Pregnancy-related. Ectopic pregnancy, abortion

Hormonal contraception

Hypothalamic-related. Chronic or systemic illness, stress, athletics, eating disorder, obesity, drugs

Pituitary-related. Prolactinoma

Outflow tract-related. Trauma, foreign body, vaginal tumor, cervical carcinoma, polyp, uterine myoma, uterine carcinoma, intrauterine device

Androgen excess. Chronic anovulatory hyperandrogenism (PCO), adrenal tumor, ovarian tumor, adrenal hyperplasia (classic and nonclassic)

Other endocrine causes. Thyroid disease, adrenal disease

Hematologic-related. Thrombocytopenia, abnormalities of clotting factors, abnormalities of platelet function, anticoagulant medications

Infectious causes. Pelvic inflammatory disease, cervicitis

Pelvic Pain and Ectopic Pregnancy

History: Positive pregnancy test, missed menstrual period, pelvic or abdominal pain (bilateral or unilateral), symptoms of pregnancy; abnormal uterine bleeding. Menstrual and obstetrical history.

Characteristics of pelvic pain; onset, duration; palliative or aggravating factors, shoulder pain. Rupture of ectopic pregnancy usually occurs 6-12 weeks after last menstrual period.

Associated Symptoms: Fever, vaginal discharge. Urinary or gastrointestinal symptoms, fever, abnormal bleeding, or vaginal discharge.

Past Medical History: Surgical history, gynecologic history, sexually transmitted diseases.

Method of Contraception: Oral contraceptives or barrier method, intrauterine device (IUD). Current sexual activity and practices.

Risk Factors for Ectopic Pregnancy: Prior pelvic infection, endometriosis, prior ectopic pregnancy, pelvic tumor, intrauterine device, pelvic/tubal surgery, infertility, diethylstilbestrol exposure in utero.

Physical Exam

General: Moderate to severe distress.

Vitals: BP (orthostatic hypotension), P (tachycardia), R, T (low fever).

Skin: Cold clammy skin, pallor.

Abdomen: Cullen's sign (periumbilical darkening, intra abdominal bleeding), local then generalized tenderness, tenderness, rebound (peritoneal signs).

Pelvic: Cervical discharge, cervical motion tenderness; Chadwick's sign (cervical and vaginal cyanosis; pregnancy); Hegar's sign (softening of uterine isthmus; pregnancy); enlarged uterus; tender adnexal mass or cul-de-sac fullness.

Labs: Quantitative beta-HCG, transvaginal ultrasound. Type and hold, Rh, CBC, UA with micro; GC, chlamydia culture. Laparoscopy.

Differential Diagnosis

Pregnancy-Related Causes. Ectopic pregnancy, abortion (spontaneous, threatened, or incomplete), intrauterine pregnancy with corpus luteum bleeding.

Gynecologic Disorders. PID, endometriosis, ovarian cyst hemorrhage or rupture, adnexal torsion, Mittelschmerz, uterine leiomyoma torsion, primary dysmenorrhea, tumor.

Nonreproductive Tract Causes

    Gastrointestinal. Appendicitis, inflammatory bowel disease, mesenteric adenitis, irritable bowel syndrome, diverticulitis.

    Urinary Tract. Urinary tract infection, renal calculus.

Neurologic Disorders

Headache

History: Quality (dull, band-like, sharp, throbbing), location (retroorbital, temporal, suboccipital, bilateral or unilateral), time course of typical headache episode; onset (gradual or sudden); exacerbating or relieving factors; time of day, effect of supine posture.

Age at onset of headaches; change in severity, frequency; awakening from sleep; family history of migraine; analgesic or codeine use. "The worst headache ever" (subarachnoid hemorrhage).

Aura or Prodrome: Scotomata, blurred vision; nausea, vomiting, sensory disturbances.

Associated Symptoms: Numbness, weakness, diplopia, photophobia, fever, nasal discharge (sinusitis); neck stiffness (meningitis); eye pain or redness (glaucoma); ataxia, dysarthria, transient blindness, neck pain. Lacrimation, flushing, intermittent periodicity (cluster headaches).

Aggravating or Relieving Factors: Relief by analgesics or sleep. Exacerbation by foods (chocolate, alcohol, wine, cheese), emotional upset, menses; hypertension, trauma; lack of or excess sleep; exacerbation by fatigue, exertion, monosodium glutamate, nitrates.

Drugs: Nitrates, phenothiazines, sedatives, theophylline, sympathomimetics, estrogen, corticosteroids, excessive ergotamine, cold remedies, eye drops, diet pills, cocaine.

Symptoms of Depression: Sleep disturbance, decreased energy, loss of interest in usual pleasurable activities, poor concentration, depressed mood. Weight loss, decreased appetite.

Physical Exam

Vitals: BP (hypertension), P, T (fever), R.

HEENT: Cranial or temporal tenderness (temporal arteritis), asymmetric pupil reactivity; papilledema, extraocular movements, visual field deficits. Conjunctival injection, lacrimation, rhinorrhea (cluster headache).

Jaw or temporomandibular joint tenderness (TMJ syndrome); temporal or ocular bruits (arteriovenous malformation); sinus tenderness (sinusitis).

Dental infection, tooth tenderness to percussion (abscess); paraspinal muscle tenderness.

Neck: Neck rigidity.

Skin: Cafe au lait spots (neurofibromatosis); adenoma sebaceum (facial angiofibromas).

Neuro: Cranial nerve palsies (intracranial tumor); auditory acuity, focal weakness, tendon reflexes, ataxia.

Labs: Electrolytes, ESR, MRI scan, lumbar puncture. CBC with differential, PT/PTT.

Indications for MRI scan: Focal neurologic signs, papilledema, decreased visual acuity, increased frequency or severity of headache, excruciating or paroxysmal headache, awakening from sleep, persistent vomiting, head trauma with focal neurologic signs or lethargy.

Differential Diagnosis: Migraine, tension headache; systemic infection, subarachnoid hemorrhage, sinusitis, arteriovenous malformation, malignant hypertension, temporal arteritis, meningitis, encephalitis, post concussion syndrome, intracranial tumor, venous sinus thrombosis, benign intracranial hypertension (pseudotumor cerebri), subdural hematoma, trigeminal neuralgia, post-herpetic neuralgia, glaucoma, brain abscess, analgesic overuse, psychogenic headache.

Characteristics of Migraine: Childhood to early adult onset; usually a family history; aura of scotomas or scintillations, unilateral pulsating or throbbing pain; nausea, vomiting. Lasts 2-6 hours; relief with sleep.

Characteristics of Tension Headache: Bilateral, generalized, bitemporal or suboccipital. Band-like pressure; throbbing pain, occurs late in day; related to stress. Onset in adolescence or young adult; nonfamilial. Lasts hours and is usually relieved by simple analgesics.

Characteristics of Cluster Headache: Recurrent, unilateral, retroorbital searing pain. Lacrimation, nasal and conjunctival congestion. Young males; lasts 20-60 min. Occurs in clusters at same time of night or several times each day over several weeks; followed by pain-free periods.

Dizziness and Vertigo

History: Sensation of spinning or movement of surroundings, light headedness, nausea, vomiting, tinnitus. Rate of onset and intensity of vertigo. Aggravation by change in position, turning of head, changing from supine to standing, coughing.

Hyperventilation, postural unsteadiness. Recent change in eyeglasses. Headache, hearing loss, head trauma.

Associated Symptoms: Recent upper respiratory infection, diplopia, paresthesias, syncope; hypertension, diabetes, history of stroke, transient ischemic attack, anemia, cardiovascular disease.

Drugs Associated with Vertigo: Antihypertensives, aspirin, alcohol, sedatives, diuretics, phenytoin, ototoxic drugs (gentamicin, neomycin).

Physical Exam

General: Hyperventilation may provoke symptoms. Affect of Valsalva maneuver on symptoms.

Vitals: P, BP (supine and upright, postural hypotension), R, T.

HEENT: Nystagmus, visual acuity, visual field deficits, papilledema; facial weakness. Tympanic membrane inflammation (otitis media), cerumen. Effect of head turning, or of placing the patient recumbent with head extended over edge of bed; Rinne's test (air/bone conduction); Weber test (lateralization of sound).

Heart: Rhythm, murmurs.

Neuro: Cranial nerves 2-12, sensory deficits, ataxia, weakness. Romberg test, coordination (finger to nose test), tandem gait.

Rectal: Occult blood.

Labs: CBC, electrolytes, MRI scan.

Differential Diagnosis

Drugs Associated with Vertigo: Aminoglycosides, loop diuretics, aspirin, caffeine, alcohol, phenytoin, psychotropics (lithium, haloperidol), benzodiazepines.

Peripheral Causes of Vertigo: Acute labyrinthitis/neuronitis, benign positional vertigo, Meniere's disease (vertigo, tinnitus, deafness), otitis media, acoustic neuroma, cerebellopontine angle tumor, cholesteatoma (chronic middle ear effusion), impacted cerumen.

Central Causes of Vertigo: Vertebrobasilar insufficiency, brain stem or cerebellar infarctions, tumors, encephalitis, meningitis, brain stem or cerebellar contusion, Parkinson's disease, multiple sclerosis.

Other Disorders Associated with Vertigo: Motion sickness, presyncope, syndrome of multiple sensory deficits (peripheral neuropathies, visual impairment, orthopedic problems), altered visual input (new eyeglasses), orthostatic hypotension.

Delirium, Coma, and Confusion

History: Level of consciousness, obtundation (awake but not alert), stupor (unconscious but awakable with vigorous stimulation), coma (cannot be awakened). Confusion, hallucination, delirium, tremor, poor concentration, agitations.

Activity and symptoms prior to onset. Use of insulin, oral hypoglycemics, narcotics, alcohol, drugs, antipsychotics, anticholinergics, anticoagulants; history of trauma, suicide attempts or depression, prior epilepsy (post-ictal state).

Fever, headache, history of dementia, stroke, transient ischemic attacks, hypertension; renal, liver or cardiac disease.

Physical Exam

General: Signs of dehydration.

Vitals: BP (hypertensive encephalopathy), P, T (fever), R.

HEENT: Skull palpation for tenderness, lacerations. Pupil size and reactivity; extraocular movements, corneal reflexes. Papilledema, hemorrhages, flame lesions; facial asymmetry, ptosis, weakness. Battle's sign (ecchymosis over mastoid process), raccoon sign (periorbital ecchymosis, skull fracture), hemotympanum (basal skull fracture). Tongue or cheek lacerations (post-ictal state). Signs of B12 deficiency (atrophic tongue).

Neck: Neck rigidity, carotid bruits.

Chest: Breathing pattern (Cheyne-Stokes hyperventilation); crackles, wheezes.

Heart: Rhythm, murmurs.

Abdomen: Hepatomegaly, splenomegaly, masses, ascites, tenderness, distention, dilated superficial veins (liver failure).

Extremities: Track marks (drug overdose).

Skin: Cyanosis, jaundice, spider angiomata, palmar erythema (hepatic encephalopathy); capillary refill, petechia, splinter hemorrhages. Localized fat atrophy (diabetes).

Neuro: Concentration (subtraction of serial 7's, delirium), strength, cranial nerves 2-12, mini-mental status exam; orientation to person, place, time, recent events; coordination, Babinski's sign, primitive reflexes (snout, suck, glabella, palmomental grasp). Tremor (Parkinson's disease, delirium tremens), incoherent speech, lethargy, somnolence.

Glasgow Coma Scale

Best Verbal Response: None - 1; incomprehensible sounds or cries - 2;

appropriate words or vocal sounds - 3; confused speech or words - 4; oriented speech - 5

Best Eye Opening Response: No eye opening - 1; eyes open to pain - 2; eyes open to speech - 3; eyes open spontaneously - 4

Best Motor Response: None - 1; abnormal extension to pain - 2; abnormal flexion to pain - 3; withdraws to pain - 4; localizes to pain - 5; obeys commands - 6

Total Possible Score: 3-15

Special Neurologic Signs

Decortication: Painful stimuli causes flexion of arms, wrist and fingers with leg extension; indicates damage to contralateral hemisphere above midbrain.

Decerebration: Painful stimuli causes extension of legs and arms; wrists and fingers flex; indicates midbrain and pons functioning.

Oculocephalic Reflex (Doll's eyes maneuver): Eye movements in response to lateral rotation of head; no eye movements or loose movements occurs in bihemispheric (diencephalon) lesion.

Oculovestibular Reflex (Cold caloric maneuver): Raise head 60 degrees and irrigate ear with cold water; causes tonic deviation of eyes to irrigated ear if intact brain stem; if the patient is conscious, it causes nystagmus, vertigo, and/or emesis.

Labs: Glucose, electrolytes, calcium, BUN, creatinine, ABG. CT/MRI, ammonia, alcohol, liver function tests, urine toxicology screen, B-12, folate levels. LP if no signs of elevated intracranial pressure and suspicion of meningitis.

Differential Diagnosis of Delirium: Electrolyte imbalance, hyperglycemia, hypoglycemia (insulin overdose), alcohol or drug withdraw or intoxication, hypoxia, meningitis, encephalitis, systemic infection, stroke, intracranial hemorrhage, postictal state, exacerbation of dementia; narcotic or anticholinergic overdose; steroid withdrawal, hepatic encephalopathy; psychotic states, dehydration, hypertensive encephalopathy, head trauma, subdural hematoma, uremia, vitamin B12 or folate deficiency, hypothyroidism, ketoacidosis, factitious coma.

Weakness and Ischemic Stroke

History: Rate and pattern of onset of weakness (gradual, sudden); time of onset and time course to maximum deficit; anatomic location of deficit; activity prior to onset (Valsalva, exertion, neck movement, sleeping); improvement or progression of symptoms; headache prior to event, nausea, vomiting, loss of consciousness; visual aura, vertigo, seizure.

Confusion, dysarthria, incontinence, dysphagia, palpitations; prior transient ischemic attacks (neurologic deficit lasting less than 24 hours) or strokes; past transient monocular blindness (Amaurosis fugax).

Past Medical History: Hypertension, diabetes, coronary disease, endocarditis, hyperlipidemia, IV drug abuse, cocaine use, heart failure, valvular disease, arrhythmias (atrial fibrillation), claudication, anticoagulants, alcohol, antihypertensives, cigarette smoking.

Past testing: CT scans, carotid Doppler studies, echocardiograms.

Family history: Stroke, hyperlipidemia, cardiac disease.

Physical Exam

General: Level of consciousness, lethargy.

Vitals: BP (both arms), P (bradycardia), T, R. Cushing's response (bradycardia, hypertension, abnormal respirations).

HEENT: Signs of head trauma, pupil size and reactivity, extraocular movements. Fundi: hypertensive retinopathy, Roth spots (flame shaped lesions, endocarditis), subhyaloid retinal hemorrhages (blood pocket indicating subarachnoid hemorrhage), papilledema; facial asymmetry or weakness.

Neck: Neck rigidity, carotid bruits.

Chest: Breathing pattern, Cheyne Stokes respiration (periodic breathing with periods of apnea, elevated intracranial pressure).

Heart: Irregular, irregular rhythm (atrial fibrillation), S3 (heart failure), murmurs (mitral stenosis, cardiogenic emboli).

Abdomen: Aortic pulsations, renal bruits (atherosclerotic disease).

Extremities: Unequal peripheral pulses.

Skin: Petechia, splinter hemorrhages.

Neuro: Focal motor deficits, gag reflex, cranial nerves 2-12, gaze, ptosis, Babinski's sign (stroke sole of foot, and toes dorsiflex if pyramidal tract lesion). Clonus, primitive reflexes (snout, glabella, palmomental, grasp). Mini-mental status exam, memory concentration.

Signs of Increased Intracranial Pressure: Lethargy, headache, vomiting, meningismus, papilledema, focal neurologic deficits.

Signs of Cerebral Herniation: Obtundation, dilation of ipsilateral pupil, decerebrate posturing (extension of elbows, wrists and legs), ascending weakness. Cushing's response - bradycardia, hypertension, abnormal respirations.

Labs: CT scan: bleeding, infarction, mass effect, midline shift. ECG, CBC.

Differential Diagnosis of Stroke Syndromes: Infection (abscess, meningitis, encephalitis), subdural hematoma, brain tumor, metabolic imbalance (hypoglycemia, hypocalcemia), vasculitis, postictal paralysis (Todd's paralysis), delirium; conversion reaction; atypical migraine, basilar artery stenosis, transient ischemic attack.

Seizure

History: Time of onset of seizure, duration of seizure, type (tonic-clonic), description of seizure. Past seizures, noncompliance with anticonvulsant medication (recent blood level). Aura (irritability, behavioral change, lethargy), pallor, incontinence of urine or feces, vomiting, post-ictal weakness or paralysis.

Prodrome (visual changes, paresthesias), stroke, migraine headaches, fever, chills. Diabetes (hypoglycemia), family history of epilepsy.

Factors that May Precipitate Seizures: Fatigue, sleep deprivation, infection, hyperventilation, head trauma, alcohol or drug withdrawal, cocaine intoxication; meningitis, high fever, uremia, hypoglycemia, theophylline toxicity, stroke.

Past testing: EEG's, CT scans.

Physical Exam

General: Post-ictal lethargy.

Vitals: BP (hypertension), P, R, T (hyperpyrexia).

HEENT: Evidence of head trauma; pupil reactivity and equality, extraocular movements; papilledema, gum hyperplasia (phenytoin); tongue or buccal lacerations; carotid bruits, neck rigidity.

Chest: Rhonchi, wheeze (aspiration).

Heart: Rhythm, murmurs.

Extremities: Cyanosis, fractures.

Genitourinary/Rectal: Incontinence of urine or feces.

Skin: Café-au-lait spots, neurofibromas (Von Recklinghausen's disease), splinter hemorrhages (endocarditis). Unilateral port-wine facial nevus (Sturge-Weber syndrome); facial angiofibromas (adenoma sebaceum), hypopigmented ash leaf spots (tuberous sclerosis). Spider angiomas (hepatic encephalopathy).

Neuro: Dysarthria, sensory deficits, visual field deficits, focal weakness (Todd's paralysis), cranial nerves, Babinski's sign.

Labs: Glucose, electrolytes, calcium, liver function tests, CBC, urine toxicology, anticonvulsant levels, RPR/VDRL. EEG, MRI, lumbar puncture.

Differential Diagnosis: Epilepsy (complex partial seizure disorder, generalized seizure disorder), noncompliance with anticonvulsant medications, hypoglycemia, hyponatremia, hypocalcemia, hypomagnesemia, hypertensive encephalopathy, alcohol withdrawal, meningitis, encephalitis, brain tumor, stroke, vasculitis, pseudo-seizure.

Renal Disorders

Oliguria, Anuria, and Acute Renal Failure

History: Oliguria (<20 mL/h, 400-500 mL urine/day); anuria (<100 mL urine/day); hemorrhage, heart failure, sepsis, infection, vomiting, nasogastric suction; diarrhea, fever, chills; measured fluid input and output by Foley catheter; prostate enlargement, kidney stones, anticholinergics.

Nephrotoxic drugs (aminoglycosides, neomycin, amphotericin, NSAID's), dysuria, flank pain. Abdominal pain; hematuria, passing of tissue fragments, foamy urine (proteinuria). Administration of renally excreted medications.

Recent upper respiratory infection (post streptococcal glomerulonephritis), recent chemotherapy (tumor lysis syndrome).

Physical Exam

Vitals: BP (orthostatic vitals; an increase in heart rate by >15 mmHg and a fall in systolic pressure >15 mmHg, indicates significant volume depletion); P (tachycardia); T (fever), R (tachypnea).

Skin: Decreased skin turgor over sternum (hypovolemia); skin temperature and color; jaundice (hepatorenal syndrome).

HEENT: Oral mucous membrane moisture, ocular moisture, flat neck veins (volume depletion), venous distention (heart failure).

Chest: Crackles (heart failure).

Heart: S3 (volume overload).

Abdomen: Hepatomegaly, abdominojugular reflex (heart failure); costovertebral angle tenderness; distended bladder, nephromegaly (obstruction).

Pelvic: Pelvic masses, cystocele, urethrocele.

Rectal: Prostate hypertrophy; absent sphincter reflex and decreased sensation (atonic bladder due to vertebral disk herniation).

Extremities: Peripheral edema (heart failure).

Labs: Sodium, potassium, BUN, creatinine, uric acid. Urine and serum osmolality, UA, urine creatinine. Ultrasound of bladder and kidneys.

Fractional excretion of sodium (FE Na) = $\dfrac{U_{Na}(mMol/L) \times S_{Cr}(mMol/L)}{S_{Na}(mMol/L) \; U_{Cr}(mMol/L)} \times 100$

Renal Failure Index = $\dfrac{UNa \times 100}{U/PCr}$

Clinical Findings in Pre-renal, Renal, Post-renal Failure			
	Prerenal	**ARF**	**Postrenal**
BUN/Creatinine ratio	>15:1	<15:1	varies
Urine sodium	<20 mMol/L	>20	varies
Urine osmolality	>500 mOsm/kg	<350	varies
Renal failure Index	<1	>1	varies
FE Na	<1%	>1%	varies
Urine/plasma creatinine	>40	>20	varies
Urine analyses	normal	cellular casts	RBC's, WBC's, bacteria

Differential Diagnosis of Acute Renal Failure
Prerenal Insult
  A. Prerenal insult is the most common cause of acute renal failure, accounting for 70%.
  B. It is usually caused by reduced renal perfusion pressure secondary to extracellular fluid volume loss (diarrhea, diuresis, GI hemorrhage), or secondary to extracellular fluid sequestration (pancreatitis, sepsis), inadequate cardiac output, renal vasoconstriction (sepsis, liver disease, drugs), or inadequate fluid intake or replacement.
Intrarenal Insult
  A. Insult to the renal parenchyma (tubular necrosis) causes 20% of acute renal failure.
  B. Prolonged hypoperfusion is the most common cause of tubular necrosis.
  C. Nephrotoxins (radiographic, aminoglycosides, contrast) are the second

most common cause of tubular necrosis. Less common nephrotoxins include cisplatin, amphotericin, and pentamidine.

D. Pigmenturia induced renal injury can be caused by intravascular hemolysis or rhabdomyolysis.

E. Other causes of tubular necrosis include pyelonephritis, thrombosis, emboli, malignant hypertension, thrombotic thrombocytopenic purpura, hemolytic-uremic syndrome, and vasculitis.

F. Acute glomerulonephritis or acute inflammation of renal interstitium (acute interstitial nephritis) (usually from allergic reactions to beta-lactam antibiotics, sulfonamides, rifampin, NSAIDs, cimetidine, phenytoin, allopurinol, thiazides, furosemide, analgesics) are occasional causes of intrarenal kidney failure.

Postrenal Insult

A. Postrenal damage results from obstruction of urine flow, and it is the least common cause of acute renal failure, accounting for 10%.

B. Postrenal insult may be caused by extrarenal obstructive uropathy (prostate cancer, benign prostatic hypertrophy, renal calculi obstruction) or by intrarenal obstruction of the distal tubules (amyloidosis, uric acid crystals, multiple myeloma, methotrexate, or acyclovir).

Chronic Renal Failure

History: Oliguria, current and baseline creatinine, and BUN. Diabetes, hypertension; history of pyelonephritis, sepsis, heart failure, liver disease, peripheral edema; dark colored urine, rashes or purpura; medications (nonsteroidal anti-inflammatory drugs, aminoglycosides, contrast dyes). Hypovolemia secondary to diarrhea, hemorrhage, over-diuresis; glomerulonephritis, interstitial nephritis.

Past ultrasounds, flank pain, history of kidney stones, prostate disease, urethral obstruction. Anorexia, insomnia, fatigue, malaise, weight loss, bleeding diathesis, paresthesias, anemia.

History of pathologic fractures, family history of polycystic kidney disease, hereditary glomerulonephritis.

Physical Exam

General: Evaluate intravascular volume status.

Vitals: Postural blood pressure and pulse (tachycardia, hypertension), T (fever), R.

Skin: Skin turgor, sallow yellow skin (urochromes), fine white powder (uremic frost), purpura, petechiae (coagulopathy). Jaundice, spider angiomas (hepatorenal syndrome).

HEENT: Neck vein distention (volume overload).

Chest: Crackles (rales).

Heart: S3 gallop (volume overload), cardiac friction rub (pericarditis), displacement of heart border, muffled heart sounds (effusion), arrhythmias (electrolyte imbalances).

Abdomen: Distended bladder, costovertebral angle or suprapubic tenderness, pelvic masses, ascites.

Rectal: Occult blood, prostate enlargement.

Neuro: Asterixis, myoclonus, decreased sensation.

Labs: BUN, creatinine, potassium (hyperkalemia), albumin, lipids, calcium, phosphorus, proteinuria.

Differential Diagnosis of Chronic Renal Failure: Hypertensive nephrosclerosis, diabetic nephrosclerosis, glomerulonephritis, polycystic kidney disease, tubulointerstitial renal disease, reflux nephropathy, analgesic nephropathy, chronic obstructive uropathy, amyloidosis, Lupus nephropathy.

Hematuria

History: Frequency, dysuria, suprapubic pain, flank pain (renal colic), abdominal or perineal pain; fever. Recent exercise, menstruation; bleeding between voidings.

Foley catheterization, prior stones, tissue passage in urine, joint pain.

Color, timing, pattern of hematuria: Initial hematuria (anterior urethral lesion); terminal hematuria (bladder neck or prostate lesion); hematuria throughout voiding (bladder or upper urinary tract).

Recent sore throat, streptococcal skin infection (glomerulonephritis). Prior pyelonephritis, joint pain; occupational exposure to toxins.

Family History: Hematuria, renal disease, sickle cell, bleeding diathesis, deafness (Alport's syndrome), hypertension.

Medications Associated with Hematuria: Warfarin, aspirin, ibuprofen, naproxen, phenobarbital, allopurinol, phenytoin, cyclophosphamide.

Causes of Red Urine: Pyridium, phenytoin, ibuprofen, chloroquine, cascara laxatives, levodopa, methyldopa, quinine, rifampin, berries, flava beans, food coloring, rhubarb, beets, hemoglobinuria, myoglobinuria.

Physical Exam

Vitals: BP (hypertension).

Skin: Rashes.

HEENT: Pharyngitis, carotid bruits.

Heart: Heart murmur; irregular, irregular (atrial fibrillation, renal emboli).

Abdomen: Tenderness, masses, costovertebral angle tenderness (renal calculus or pyelonephritis), abdominal bruits, nephromegaly, suprapubic tenderness.

Genitourinary: Urethral lesions, discharge, condyloma, foreign body, cervical malignancy; prostate tenderness, nodules, or enlargement (prostatitis, prostate cancer).

Extremities: Peripheral edema (nephrotic syndrome), arthritis, ecchymoses, petechiae, weak or unequal peripheral pulses (aortic dissection).

Labs: UA with microscopic exam of urinary sediment, CBC, KUB, intravenous pyelogram, ultrasound. Streptozyme panel, ANA, PT/PTT.

Indicators of Significant Hematuria: (1) >3 RBC's per high-power field on 2 of 3 specimens; (2) >100 RBC's per HPF in 1 specimen; (3) gross hematuria
The patient should abstain from exercise for 48 hours prior to urine collection, and it should not be collected during menses.

Differential Diagnosis

    A. Medical Hematuria is caused by a glomerular lesion; plasma proteins filter into urine out of proportion to the amount of hematuria. It is characterized by glomerular RBC's that are distorted with crenated membranes and an uneven hemoglobin distribution and casts. Microscopic hematuria and a urine dipstick test of 2+ protein is more likely to have a medical cause.

    B. Urologic Hematuria is caused by a urologic lesion such as a urinary stone or carcinoma; it is characterized by minimal proteinuria, and protein appears in urine proportional to the amount of whole blood present. Non-glomerular RBC's (disk shaped with an even hemoglobin distribution) and absence of casts are characteristic.

Nephrolithiasis

History: Severe, colicky, intermittent, migrating, lower abdominal pain; flank pain, hematuria, fever, dysuria; prior history of renal stones. Pain is not associated with position; abdominal pain may radiate laterally around abdomen to groin, testicles or labia. History of low fluid intake, urinary tract infection.

Excessive calcium administration, immobilization, furosemide, neurogenic bladder, chemotherapy; family history of kidney stones. Inflammatory bowel disease, ileal resection. Diet high in oxalate: Spinach, rhubarb, nuts, tea, cocoa. Excess vitamin C intake, hydrochlorothiazide; unusual dietary habits.

Physical Exam Costovertebral angle tenderness, suprapubic tenderness; enlarged kidney.

Labs: Serum calcium, phosphorus, bicarbonate, creatinine, uric acid. Urine cystine, UA microscopic (hematuria), urine culture, intravenous pyelogram.

Differential Diagnosis: Nephrolithiasis, cystitis, diverticulitis, appendicitis, salpingitis, torsion of hernia, ovarian torsion, ovarian cyst rupture or hemorrhage, bladder obstruction, prostatitis, prostate cancer, endometriosis, ectopic pregnancy, colonic obstruction, inflammatory bowel disease, carcinoma (colon, prostrate, cervix, bladder).

Causes of Nephrolithiasis: Hypercalcemia, hyperuricosuria, hyperoxaluria, cystinuria, distal renal tubular acidosis (type 1), Proteus mirabilis urinary tract infection with staghorn calculi.

Hyperkalemia

History: Serum potassium >5.5 mMol/L (repeat test to exclude lab error); muscle weakness, syncope, lightheadedness, palpitations, oliguria; excess intake of oral or intravenous potassium, salt substitutes, potassium sparing diuretics, angiotensin converting enzyme inhibitors; nonsteroidal anti-inflammatory drugs, beta blockers, heparin, digoxin toxicity; muscle trauma, chemotherapy (tumor lysis syndrome), cyclosporine, succinylcholine.

History of renal disease, diabetes, adrenal insufficiency (Addison's syndrome). History of episodic paralysis precipitated by exercise (familial hyperkalemic periodic paralysis).

Physical Exam

Skin: Hyperpigmentation (Addison's disease), hematomas.

Abdomen: Suprapubic tenderness.

Neuro: Muscle weakness, abnormal deep tendon reflexes, cranial nerves 2-12.

Labs: Potassium, platelets, bicarbonate, chloride, anion gap, LDH, bilirubin, urine K, pH. Serum aldosterone, plasma renin activity.

ECG: Tall peaked, precordial T waves; diminished QT interval; widened QRS complex, prolonged PR interval, P wave flattening, AV block, ventricular arrhythmias, sine wave, asystole.

Differential Diagnosis
Inadequate Excretion: Renal failure, adrenal insufficiency (Addison's syndrome), potassium sparing diuretics (spironolactone), urinary tract obstruction, lupus, hypoaldosteronism, ACE inhibitors, NSAIDs, heparin.
Increased Potassium Production: Hemolysis, rhabdomyolysis, muscle crush injury, internal hemorrhage, drugs (succinylcholine, digoxin overdose, beta blockers), acidosis, hyperkalemic periodic paralysis, hyperosmolality.
Excess Intake of Potassium: Oral or IV potassium supplements, salt substitutes.
Pseudo-hyperkalemia: Hemolysis after collection of blood, use of excessively small needle, excessive shaking of sample, delayed transport of blood to lab, thrombocytosis, leukocytosis, prolonged tourniquet use while drawing blood.

Hypokalemia

History: Potassium <3.5 mMol/L (repeat test to exclude lab error), hyperglycemia, diuretics, diarrhea, vomiting, laxative abuse; poor intake of potassium containing foods; corticosteroids, nephrotoxins, bicarbonate, beta agonists. Conn's syndrome (hyperaldosteronism).
Associated Symptoms: Muscle weakness, cramping pain, nausea, vomiting, constipation, palpitations, paresthesias, paralysis, polyuria.
Precipitating Factors: Renal disease, stress (catecholamine release), cellular proliferation (Vitamin B12 treatment); biliary drainage, enteric fistula; Kayexalate ingestion, dialysis, excessive licorice ingestion, chewing tobacco.

Physical Exam
Vitals: BP, P, T, R.
Heart: Rate and rhythm.
Abdomen: Hypoactive bowel sounds (ileus).
Neuro: Weakness, hypoactive tendon reflexes.
Labs: Serum potassium. 24 hour urine potassium >20 mEq/day indicates

excessive urinary K loss. If <20 mEq/d, low K intake or nonurinary K loss is the cause. Electrolytes, BUN, creatinine, glucose, magnesium, CBC, plasma renin activity, aldosterone. Urine specific gravity, osmolality.

ECG: Flattening and inversion of T-waves (II, V3), ST segment depression, U waves (II, V1, V2, V3); first or second degree block, QT interval prolongation, premature atrial or ventricular contractions, supraventricular tachycardia, ventricular tachycardia or fibrillation.

Differential Diagnosis of Hypokalemia

Cellular Redistribution of Potassium: Intracellular shift of potassium by insulin (exogenous or glucose load), beta2 agonist; stress induced catecholamine release, thyrotoxic periodic paralysis; alkalosis-induced shift (metabolic or respiratory); familial periodic paralysis, cellular proliferation (vitamin B12 treatment), hypothermia; acute myeloid leukemia.

Nonrenal Potassium Loss:

> **Gastrointestinal Loss.** Diarrhea, laxative abuse, villous adenoma, biliary drainage, enteric fistula, potassium binding resin ingestion

> **Non-gastrointestinal Loss.** Sweating, prolonged low potassium ingestion, dialysis

Renal Potassium Loss:

> **Hypertensive High Renin States.** Malignant hypertension, renal artery stenosis, renin-producing tumor.

> **Hypertensive Low Renin, High Aldosterone States.** Primary hyperaldosteronism (adenoma or hyperplasia).

> **Hypertensive Low Renin, Low Aldosterone States.** Congenital adrenal hyperplasia, Cushing's syndrome, exogenous mineralocorticoids (Florinef, licorice, chewing tobacco), Liddle's syndrome

> **Normotensive.** Renal tubular acidosis (type I or II), metabolic alkalosis with a urine Cl <10 mEq/day is caused by vomiting; metabolic alkalosis with a urine Cl >10 mEq/day is caused by Bartter's syndrome, diuretics, magnesium depletion, normotensive hyperaldosteronism

Hyponatremia

History: Serum sodium <135 mMol/L; decreased mental status, confusion, agitation, irritability, lethargy, anorexia, nausea, vomiting, headache, muscle weakness or tremor, cramps, seizures; decreased output of dark urine (dehydration); polydipsia (water intoxication); diuretics, diarrhea, steroid withdrawal.

Renal, CNS, or pulmonary disease (syndrome of inappropriate antidiuretic hormone); heart failure, cirrhosis; hypotonic IV fluids, psychotropic medications, chemotherapeutic agents, hyperalimentation, hypothyroidism. Low sodium diet, hyperlipidemia (pseudohyponatremia).

Physical Exam

Vitals: BP, P (orthostatic vitals), T, R.

Skin: Decreased skin turgor, delayed capillary refill; hyperpigmentation (Addison's disease), moon-face, truncal obesity (hypocortisolism with steroid withdrawal).

HEENT: Decreased ocular and oral moisture.

Chest: Cheyne-Stokes respirations, crackles.

Heart: Rhythm and rate. Premature ventricular contractions.

Abdomen: Ascites, tenderness.

Extremities: Edema.

Neuro: Confusion, irritability, motor weakness, ataxia, positive Babinski's sign, muscle twitches; hypoactive deep tendon reflexes, cranial nerve palsies.

Labs: Electrolytes, BUN, creatinine, cholesterol, triglycerides, glucose, protein, osmolality, albumin; CXR, ECG.

Differential Diagnosis of Hyponatremia Based on Urine Osmolality

    A. Low Urine Osmolality (50-180 mOsm/L). Primary excessive water intake (psychogenic water drinking).

    B. High Urine Osmolality (urine osmolality >serum osmolality)

        1. **High Urine Sodium (>40 mEq/L) and Volume Contracted.** Renal fluid loss (excessive diuretic use, salt-wasting nephropathy, Addison's disease, osmotic diuresis).

        2. **High Urine Sodium (>40 mEq/L) and Normal Volume.** Water retention caused by a drug (carbamazepine, cyclophosphamide), hypothyroidism, syndrome of inappropriate antidiuretic hormone secretion.

3. **Low Urine Sodium (<20 mEq/L) and Volume Contraction.** Extrarenal source of fluid loss (vomiting, burns).
4. **Low Urine Sodium (<20 mEq/L) and Volume-expanded, Edematous.** Heart failure, cirrhosis with ascites, nephrotic syndrome.

Hypernatremia

History: Serum sodium >145 mEq/L. History of dehydration due to fever, vomiting, burns, heat exposure, diarrhea, severely elevated glucose, salt ingestion, administration of hypertonic fluids (sodium bicarbonate, sodium chloride), sweating, impaired access to water, adipsia (lack of thirst); head injury.

Altered mental status, lethargy, agitation, polyuria, anorexia, muscle twitching, renal disease. Recent fluid intake.

Drugs causing hypernatremia: Amphotericin, phenytoin, lithium, aminoglycosides.

Physical Exam

General: Lethargy, obtundation, stupor.

Vitals: BP (orthostatic hypotension), P (tachycardia), T, R; decreased urine output.

Skin: Decreased skin turgor ("doughy" consistency), delayed capillary refill, hyperpigmentation (Conn's syndrome), moon-face, truncal obesity, stria (hypoadrenal crisis, steroid withdrawal).

HEENT: Dry mucous membranes, flat neck veins, decreased eye turgor.

Neuro: Decreased muscle tone, ataxia, tremor, hyperreflexia; extensor plantar reflexes (Babinski's sign), tonic spasms, spasticity.

Labs: Increased hematocrit; sodium, BUN, creatinine, urine and serum, osmolality. Spot urine sodium, creatinine.

Differential Diagnosis:

Hypernatremia with Hypovolemia

A. **Extrarenal Loss of Water (urine sodium >20 mMol/L).** Vomiting, diarrhea, sweating, pancreatitis, respiratory water loss.

B. **Renal loss of water (urine sodium <10 mMol/L).** diuretics, hyperglycemia, renal failure.

Euvolemic Hypernatremia Renal Water Losses. Diabetes insipidus (central or nephrogenic secretion of excessive antidiuretic hormone).

Hypernatremia with Hypervolemia (urine sodium >20 mMol/L): Hypertonic solutions of sodium chloride or bicarbonate, hyperaldosteronism, Cushing's, syndrome, congenital adrenal hyperplasia.

Endocrinologic Disorders

Diabetic Ketoacidosis

History: Initial glucose level, ketones, anion gap. Polyuria, polyphagia, polydipsia, fatigue, lethargy, nausea, vomiting, weight loss; noncompliance with insulin, hypoglycemic agents, or diet; blurred vision, physical stress, infection, dehydration, abdominal pain, dyspnea.

Cough, fever, chills, ear pain (otitis media), dysuria, frequency (urinary tract infection); back, chest or abdominal pain; frequent Candida albicans or bacterial infections.

Factors that May Precipitate Diabetic Ketoacidosis. New onset of diabetes, noncompliance with insulin, acute illness (infection, pancreatitis, myocardial infarction), stress, trauma, stroke, pregnancy.

Renal disease, gastroparesis, prior ketoacidosis, decreased sensation in extremities (diabetic neuropathy), retinopathy, hypertension.

Physical Exam
General: Decreased level of consciousness. Kussmaul respirations (deep sighing breathing).
Vitals: BP (orthostatic hypotension), P (tachycardia), T (fever or hypothermia), R (tachypnea).
Skin: Decreased turgor, delayed capillary refill; hyperpigmented atrophic macules on legs (shin spots); intertriginous candidiasis, erythrasma, localized fat atrophy (insulin injections).
HEENT: Diabetic retinopathy (neovascularization, hemorrhages, exudates); acetone breath odor (musty, apple-like odor), decreased visual acuity, low oral moisture (dehydration) tympanic membrane inflammation (otitis media); flat neck veins, neck rigidity.
Chest: Rales, rhonchi.
Abdomen: Hypoactive bowel sounds (ileus), gastric dilation (gastroparesis); tenderness, costovertebral angle tenderness, suprapubic tenderness (urinary tract infection).
Extremities: Decreased pulses, foot ulcers, cellulitis.
Neuro: Delirium, confusion, peripheral neuropathy (decreased proprioception in feet), hypotonia, hyporeflexia.
Labs: Glucose, sodium, potassium, bicarbonate, chloride, BUN, creatinine, anion gap; triglycerides, phosphate, CBC, serum ketones; UA (proteinuria,

ketones). CXR, ECG.

Differential Diagnosis

 Ketosis-Causing Conditions. Alcoholic ketoacidosis or starvation.

 Acidosis-Causing Conditions

  Increased Anion Gap Acidoses. DKA, lactic acidosis, uremia, and salicylate or methanol poisoning.

  Non-Anion Gap Acidoses. Renal or gastrointestinal bicarbonate losses due to diarrhea or renal tubular acidosis.

 Hyperglycemia-Causing Conditions. Hyperosmolar nonketotic coma.

Diagnostic Criteria for DKA. Glucose ≥ 250, pH <7.3, bicarbonate <15, ketone positive $>1{:}2$ dilutions.

Hypothyroidism and Myxedema Coma

History: Lethargy, cold intolerance, constipation, weight gain or inability to lose weight, muscle weakness; thyroid swelling or mass; decreased exercise tolerance, dyspnea on exertion; mental slowing, dry hair and skin, deepening of voice; carpal tunnel syndrome, amenorrhea.

Past history of hyperthyroidism, thyroid testing, thyroid surgery or radioactive iodine treatment, antithyroid medication; lithium, amiodarone.

Somnolence, apathy, emotional lability, depression.

Myxedema madness: Agitation, disorientation, delusions, hallucinations, paranoia, restlessness, lethargy.

Family history of thyroid disease.

Factors Predisposing to Myxedema Coma. Cold exposure, infection, trauma, surgery, anesthesia, narcotics, phenothiazines, phenytoin, sedatives, propranolol, alcohol.

Physical Exam

General: Hypoactivity, confusion, somnolence, coarse, deep voice; dull, expressionless face.

Vitals: Bradycardia, hypotension, hypothermia.

Skin: Cool, dry, pale, rough, doughy skin; thin, brittle nails that are dry with longitudinal ridges; yellowish skin without scleral icterus (carotenemia). Hyperkeratosis of elbows and knees.

HEENT: Thin, dry, brittle hair, alopecia; macroglossia (enlarged tongue), puffy face and eyelids; loss of lateral third of eyebrows, thyroid enlargement, thyroid surgery scar. Jugular venous distention (pericardial effusion).

Chest: Dullness to percussion (pleural effusion).

Heart: Muffled heart sounds (pericardial effusion); displacement of lateral heart border, bradycardia.

Abdomen: Hypoactive bowel sounds (ileus), ascites (myxedematous ascites).

Extremities: Bulky muscles with diminished strength and power. Myxedema: transient local swelling after tapping a muscle.

Neuro: Hypoactive tendon reflexes with delayed return phase. Decreased mental status, stupor, ataxia; peripheral neuropathy, paresthesias, weakness.

Labs: Thyroid stimulating hormone, CBC, electrolytes, hypercholesterolemia, hypertriglyceridemia, creatinine phosphokinase, LDH.

ECG: Bradycardia, low voltage QRS complexes; flattened or inverted T waves, prolonged Q-T interval.

Differential Diagnosis of Hypothyroidism: Autoimmune thyroid disease (Hashimoto's thyroiditis, atrophic hypothyroidism), iatrogenic (thyroidectomy, radioactive iodine therapy, antithyroid medications), iodine excess or deficiency, amiodarone, lithium; hypothalamic or pituitary tumor or surgery.

Hyperthyroidism and Thyrotoxicosis

History: Tremor, nervousness, hyperkinesis (restlessness), fever, heat intolerance, irritability, palpitations, diaphoresis, insomnia; thyroid enlargement, masses, thyroid pain; oligomenorrhea, amenorrhea.

Weight loss with increased appetite; dyspnea and fatigue after slight exertion; softening of the skin; fine, silky hair texture; proximal muscle weakness (especially thighs when climbing stairs).

Palpitations, atrial fibrillation; diplopia, reduced visual acuity, eye discomfort or pain, lacrimation; recent upper respiratory infection, hyperdefecation. Previous thyroid function testing; family history of thyroid disease.

Factors Precipitating Thyroid Storm: Infection, surgery, diabetic ketoacidosis, pulmonary embolus, excess hormone medication, cerebral vascular accident, myocardial infarction, labor and delivery, iodine-131 or iodine therapy.

Physical Exam

General: Restless, anxious, hyperactive patient; delirium.

Vitals: Widened pulse pressure, hyperpyrexia (>104°F), tachycardia, hypertension.

Skin: Moist, warm, velvety skin, diaphoresis; palmar erythema, fine silky hair. Plummer's nails (distal onycholysis, separation of fingernail from nail bed), acropachy (clubbing of fingers and toes). Loss of subcutaneous fat and muscle mass.

HEENT: Exophthalmos (forward displacement of the eyeballs), proptosis, widened palpebral fissures; lid lag, infrequent blinking. Ophthalmoplegia (restricted extraocular movements), chemosis (edema of conjunctiva), conjunctival injection, corneal ulcers; periorbital edema or ecchymoses; optic nerve atrophy, impaired visual acuity, difficulty with convergence; fine tongue tremor.

Neck: Painless, diffusely enlarged, soft, rubbery thyroid without masses; thyroid thrill and bruit.

Heart: Irregular, irregular rhythm (atrial fibrillation), systolic murmur (mitral or tricuspid regurgitation, flow murmur), displacement of apical impulse. Accentuated first heart sound.

Extremities: Fine tremor; non-pitting pre-tibial edema (Grave's disease).

Neuro: Proximal muscle weakness, hyperreflexia (rapid return phase of deep tendon reflexes); rapid, pressured speech.

Labs: Thyroid tests: free T4, TSH, beta-HCG pregnancy test.

ECG: Sinus tachycardia, atrial fibrillation.

Differential Diagnosis: Grave's disease, toxic multinodular goiter, acute thyroiditis, thyrotoxicosis factitia (ingestion of thyroid hormone), trophoblastic tumor (molar pregnancy), TSH producing pituitary adenoma, postpartum thyroiditis, ectopic thyroid tissue (struma ovarii, functional follicular carcinoma), thyroid adenoma or carcinoma.

Hematologic and Rheumatologic Disorders

Deep Venous Thrombosis

History: Sudden onset of unilateral calf pain, swelling, and redness; exacerbation of pain by walking and flexing of foot, dyspnea.

Risk Factors for Deep Venous Thrombosis

    A. Venous stasis risk factors include prolonged immobilization, stroke, myocardial infarction, heart failure, obesity, varicose veins, anesthesia, age >65 years old.

    B. Endothelial injury risk factors include surgery, trauma, central venous access catheters, pacemaker wires, previous thromboembolic event.

    C. Hypercoagulable state risk factors include malignant disease, high estrogen level (pregnancy, oral contraceptives).

    D. Hematologic Disorders. Polycythemia, leukocytosis, thrombocytosis, antithrombin III deficiency, protein C deficiency, protein S deficiency, antiphospholipid syndrome, inflammatory bowel disease.

Past Medical History: Abdominal pain, peptic ulcer, melena, bleeding risk factors.

Physical Exam

Vitals: BP, P, R (tachypnea if pulmonary embolus), T (low-grade fever).

Chest: Breast masses.

Abdomen: Distention, tenderness, masses.

Genitourinary/Rectal: Occult fecal blood, prostate masses, testicular or pelvic masses, inguinal lymphadenopathy.

Extremities: >2 cm difference in calf circumference, redness, cyanosis; mottling, tenderness; Homan's sign (tenderness with dorsiflexion of foot); warmth, dilated varicose veins.

Labs: Impedance plethysmography and Doppler studies, venogram; INR/PTT, CBC, electrolytes, BUN, creatinine; ECG, UA, CXR.

Differential Diagnosis: Thrombophlebitis, ruptured Baker's cyst, lymphatic obstruction, cellulitis, muscle injury, hematoma, plantaris tendon rupture.

Connective Tissue Diseases

History: Joint pain, fatigue, malaise, weight loss, fever, skin rashes; symmetrical swelling of upper and lower extremities, morning joint stiffness, photosensitivity, muscle aches, weakness.

Hip and back pain, oral ulcers, renal disease; anemia, psychiatric illness, chest pain, dysphagia, pleurisy, positional chest pain (pericarditis), Raynaud's syndrome (red, blue or numb hands when exposed to cold); migraine headaches, stroke, depression, hypertension.

Drugs Associated with Lupus: Procainamide, isoniazid, hydralazine, methyldopa (Aldomet).

Physical Exam

Vitals: Hypertension

Skin: Skin fibrosis (thickening, scleroderma), calcinosis, telangiectasias, discoid lesions (erythematous plaques), purpura, skin ulcers, rheumatoid nodules, livedo reticularis.

HEENT: Keratoconjunctivitis sicca (dry inflammation of conjunctiva), malar rash (erythematous rash in "butterfly" pattern on the face), oral ulcers. Episcleritis or scleritis, xerophthalmia (dry eyes), parotid enlargement.

Chest: Pleural friction rub (pleuritis), fine rales (interstitial fibrosis).

Heart: Cardiac friction rubs (pericarditis).

Abdomen: Hepatosplenomegaly, abdominal tenderness.

Extremities: Joint deformities, joint tenderness, muscle weakness, lymphadenopathy sclerodactyly.

Labs: Electrolytes, creatinine, ANA, LE cell prep, VDRL, ESR, CBC, UA, ECG, complement. UA (proteinuria, casts).

Diagnostic Criteria for Rheumatoid Arthritis: Four or more of the following.
1. Morning stiffness (>6 weeks)
2. Arthritis in 3 or more joints (>6 weeks)
3. Arthritis of hand joints (>6 weeks)
4. Symmetric arthritis (>6 weeks)
5. Rheumatoid nodules
6. Positive rheumatoid factor
7. X-ray abnormalities: Erosions, bony decalcification (especially in hands/wrist).

Diagnostic Criteria for SLE: Four or more of the following.
1. Malar rash
2. Discoid rash

3. Photosensitivity
4. Oral or nasopharyngeal ulcers
5. Nonerosive arthritis
6. Pleuritis or pericarditis
7. Persistent proteinuria
8. Seizures or psychosis
9. Hemolytic anemia
10. Positive lupus erythematosus cell, positive anti-DNA antibody, Smith antibody, false positive VDRL.
11. Positive ANA

Psychiatric Disorders

Clinical Evaluation of the Psychiatric Patient

I. **Psychiatric History**
   A. **Identifying Information:** Age, sex, marital status, race.
   B. **Chief Complaint (CC):** Reason for consultation--subjective or objective; often a direct quote from the patient.
   C. **History of Present Illness (HPI)**
   1. **Current Symptoms:** Date of onset, duration and course
   2. Previous psychiatric symptoms and treatment
   3. **Recent Psychosocial Stressors:** Stressful life events which may have contributed to the patient's current presentation
   4. Reason the patient is presenting now
   5. This section should provide evidence that supports or rules out certain diagnosis.
   D. **Past Psychiatric History**
   1. Previous and current psychiatric diagnoses
   2. History of psychiatric treatment, including outpatient and inpatient treatment
   3. History of psychotropic medication use
   4. History of suicide attempts
   E. **Past Medical History**
   1. Current and/or previous medical problems
   2. Type of treatment, including prescription, over the counter medications, home or folk remedies.
   F. **Family History**: Relatives with history of psychiatric disorders, suicide or suicide attempts, alcohol or substance abuse.
   G. **Social History**
   1. Source of income
   2. Level of education, relationship history including marriages and sexual orientation, number of children; individuals that currently live with patient.
   3. Support network
   4. Current alcohol or illicit drug usage
   5. Occupational history
   H. **Developmental History**: Family structure during childhood, relation-

ships with parental figures and siblings; developmental milestones; peer relationships; school performance

II. Mental Status Exam

A. General Appearance and Behavior

1. Grooming, level of hygiene, characteristics of clothing
2. Unusual physical characteristics or movements
3. Attitude: Ability to interact with the interviewer
4. Psychomotor activity; agitation or retardation
5. Degree of eye contact

B. Affect

1. **Definition:** External range of expression observed by interviewer, most often described in terms of quality, range, and appropriateness
2. **Examples**
   a. Flat: Absence of all or most affect
   b. Blunted or restricted: moderately reduced range of affect
   c. Labile: intense changes in affect
   d. Full or wide range of affect: generally appropriate

C. Mood: Internal emotional tone of the patient as observed by the interviewer (ie, dysphoric, euphoric, angry, euthymic, anxious).

D. Thought Processes

1. Use of Language: Quality and quantity of speech
2. Rate, tone, associations and fluency of speech

E. Thought Content

1. **Definition:** Hallucinations, delusions and other perceptual disturbances
2. **Common Thought Content Disorders**
   a. **Hallucinations:** False sensory perceptions; may be auditory, visual, tactile, gustatory or olfactory in nature.
   b. **Delusions:** Fixed, false beliefs, firmly held in spite of contradictory evidence.
   c. **Illusions:** Misinterpretations of reality
   d. **Derealization:** Feelings of unrealness involving the outer environment
   e. **Depersonalization:** Feelings of unrealness, such as if one is "outside" of the body and observing his own activities
   f. **Suicidal and Homicidal Ideation:** When suicidal and homicidal ideation is present, it requires further elaboration with comments about intent and planning

F. **Cognitive Evaluation**
1. Level of consciousness
2. **Orientation:** Person, place and date
3. **Attention and Concentration:** Repeat 5 digits forwards and backwards or spell a five letter word ("world") forwards and backwards
4. **Short-Term Memory:** Ability to recall 3 objects after 5 minutes
5. **Fund of Knowledge:** Ability to name past five presidents, five large cities, or historical dates
6. **Calculations:** Subtraction of serial 7's, simple math problems
7. **Abstraction:** Proverb interpretation and similarities
G. **Insight:** Does the patient display an understanding of his current problems, and does the patient understand the implication of these problems?
H. **Judgment**
1. Ability to make sound decisions regarding everyday activities
2. Best evaluated by assessing a patient's history of decision making, rather than by asking hypothetical questions.

III. **DSM-IV Multiaxial Assessment Diagnosis**
Axis I: Clinical Disorders
Other conditions that may be a focus of clinical attention
Axis II: Personality Disorders
Mental Retardation
Axis III: General Medical Conditions
Axis IV: Psychosocial and Environmental Problems
Axis V: Global Assessment of Functioning

Mini-mental Status Exam

Orientation: What is the year, season, day of week, date, month? - 5 points
What is the state, county, city, hospital, floor ? - 5 points
Registration: Repeat 3 objects: apple, book, coat. - 3 points
Attention/Calculation: Spell "WORLD" backwards - 5 points
Memory: Recall the names of the previous 3 objects: - 3 points
Language: Name a pencil and a watch - 2 points
Repeat, "No ifs, and's or buts" - 1 point
Three stage command: "Take this paper in your right hand, fold it in half, and

put it on the floor." - 3 points
Written command: "Close your eyes." - 1 point
Write a sentence. - 1 point
Visual Spacial: Copy two overlapping pentagons - 1 point
Total Score
Normal: 25-30
Mild intellectual impairment: 20-25
Moderate intellectual impairment: 10-20
Severe intellectual impairment: 0-10

Attempted Suicide and Tricyclic Antidepressant Overdose

History: Time suicide was attempted and method. Quantity of pills; motive for attempt. Alcohol intake, other medications; place that medication was obtained; last menstrual period.

Symptoms of TCA Overdose: Dry mouth, hallucinations, seizures, agitation, visual changes.

Psychiatric History: Previous suicide attempts or threats, family support, marital conflict, alcohol or drug abuse. Availability of other dangerous medications or weapons; sources of emotional stress. Precipitating factor for suicide attempt (death, divorce, humiliating event, unemployment, medical illness); further desire to commit suicide; is there a definite plan? Was action impulsive or planned?

Detailed account of events 48-hours prior to suicide attempt and events after. Feelings of sadness, guilt, hopelessness, helplessness, persecution. Reasons that a patient has to wish to go on living. Did the patient believe that he would succeed in suicide? Is the patient upset that he is still alive? Personal or family history of emotional, physical, or sexual abuse.

Family history of depression, suicide, psychiatric disease.

Physical Exam

General: Level of consciousness, confusion, delirium; presence of potentially dangerous objects or substances (belts, shoe laces).

Vitals: BP (hypotension), P (bradycardia), T (hyperpyrexia), R.

HEENT: Signs of trauma; pupil size and reactivity, mydriasis, nystagmus.

Chest: Respiratory pattern, rhonchi (aspiration).

Heart: Rhythm (arrhythmias).

Abdomen: Decreased bowel sounds.

Extremities: Needle marks, wounds.

Neuro: Mental status exam; tremor, clonus, hyperactive reflexes.

ECG Signs of Antidepressant Overdose: QRS widening, PR or QT interval prolongation, AV block, ventricular tachycardia, Torsades de pointes vertricular arrhythmia.

Labs: Electrolytes, BUN, creatinine, glucose; ABG. Alcohol, acetaminophen levels; CXR, urine toxicology screen.

Alcohol Withdrawal

History: Alcohol intake (number of drinks per day), time of last alcohol intake; tremors, anxiety, nausea, vomiting; diaphoresis, agitation, fever, abdominal pain, headaches; hematemesis, melena, past withdrawal reactions; history of delirium tremens, blackouts, hallucinations, binge drinking, chest pain.

Past Medical History: Gastritis, ulcers, GI bleeding; hepatitis, cirrhosis, pancreatitis, drug abuse. Age of onset of heavy drinking.

Family history of alcoholism.

Physical Exam

General: Poor nutritional status, slurred speech, disorientation, diaphoresis.

Vitals: BP (hypertension), P (tachycardia), R, T (hyper/hypothermia).

HEENT: Signs of head trauma, ecchymoses. Conjunctival injection, icterus, nystagmus, extraocular movements, pupil reactivity.

Chest: Rhonchi, crackles (aspiration), gynecomastia (cirrhosis).

Heart: Rate and rhythm, murmurs.

Abdomen: Liver tenderness, hepatomegaly or liver atrophy, liver span, splenomegaly, ascites.

Genitourinary: Testicular atrophy, hernias.

Rectal: Occult blood.

Skin: Jaundice, spider angiomas (stellate arterioles with branching capillaries), palmar erythema, muscle atrophy (stigmata of liver disease).

Neuro: Cranial nerves 2-12, reflexes, ataxia. Asterixis, decreased vibratory sense (peripheral neuropathy).

Wernicke's Encephalopathy: Ophthalmoplegia, ataxia, global confusion (thiamine deficiency).

Korsakoff's Syndrome: Retrograde or antegrade amnesia, confabulation.

Labs: Electrolytes, magnesium, glucose, CBC, bilirubin, liver function tests, UA; chest X-ray; ECG.

Differential Diagnosis of Altered Mental Status: Alcohol intoxication, hypoglycemia, meningitis, drug overdose, head trauma, alcoholic ketoacidosis, anticholinergic poisoning, sedative-hypnotic withdrawal, intracranial hemorrhage.

Commonly Used Formulas

A-a gradient = $[(P_B - PH_2O) FiO_2 - PCO_2/R] - PO_2$ arterial

$= (713 \times FiO2 - pCO2/0.8) - pO2$ arterial

$P_B = 760$ mmHg; $PH_2O = 47$ mmHg ; $R \approx 0.8$
normal Aa gradient <10-15 mmHg (room air)

Arterial oxygen capacity = (Hgb(gm)/100 mL) x 1.36 mL O2/gm Hgb

Arterial O2 content = 1.36(Hgb)(SaO2)+0.003(PaO2)= NL 20 vol%

O2 delivery = CO x arterial O2 content = NL 640-1000 mL O2/min

Cardiac output = HR x stroke volume

$$CO\ L/min = \frac{125\ mL\ O2/min/M^2}{8.5\{(1.36)(Hgb)(SaO2) - (1.36)(Hgb)(SvO2)\}} \times 100$$

Normal CO = 4-6 L/min

$$SVR = \frac{MAP - CVP \times 80}{CO_{L/min}} = NL\ 800\text{-}1200\ dyne/sec/cm^2$$

$$PVR = \frac{PA - PCWP \times 80}{CO_{L/min}} = NL\ 45\text{-}120\ dyne/sec/cm^2$$

$$GFR\ mL/min = \frac{(140 - age) \times wt\ in\ Kg}{\substack{72\ (males) \times serum\ Cr\ (mg/dL) \\ 85\ (females) \times serum\ Cr\ (mg/dL)}}$$

$$Creatinine\ clearance = \frac{U\ Cr\ (mg/100\ mL) \times U\ vol\ (mL)}{P\ Cr\ (mg/100\ mL) \times time\ (1440\ min\ for\ 24h)}$$

Normal creatinine clearance = 100-125 ml/min(males), 85-105(females)

$$Body\ water\ deficit\ (L) = \frac{0.6(weight\ kg)([measured\ serum\ Na]-140)}{140}$$

$$Osmolality\ mOsm/kg = 2[Na+ K] + \frac{BUN}{2.8} + \frac{glucose}{18} = NL\ 270\text{-}290\ \frac{mOsm}{kg}$$

$$Fractional\ excreted\ Na = \frac{U\ Na/\ Serum\ Na \times 100}{U\ Cr/\ Serum\ Cr} = NL<1\%$$

Anion Gap = Na - (Cl + HCO3)

For each 100 mg/dL increase in glucose, Na+ decrease by 1.6 mEq/L.

Corrected serum Ca* (mg/dL) = measured Ca mg/dL + 0.8 x (4 - albumin g/dL)

Ideal body weight males = 50 kg for first 5 feet of height + 2.3 kg for each additional inch.

Ideal body weight females = 45.5 kg for first 5 feet + 2.3 kg for each additional inch.

Basal energy expenditure (BEE):
Males=66 + (13.7 x actual weight Kg) + (5 x height cm)-(6.8 x age)
Females= 655+(9.6 x actual weight Kg)+(1.7 x height cm)-(4.7 x age)

Nitrogen Balance = Gm protein intake/6.25 - urine urea nitrogen - (3-4 gm/d insensible loss)

Predicted Maximal Heart Rate = 220 - age

Normal ECG Intervals (sec)

PR	0.12-0.20
QRS	0.06-0.08
Heart rate/min	**Q-T**
60	0.33-0.43
70	0.31-0.41
80	0.29-0.38
90	0.28-0.36
100	0.27-0.35

Commonly Used Drug Levels

Drug	Therapeutic Range
Amikacin	Peak 25-30; trough <10 mcg/mL
Amitriptyline	100-250 ng/mL
Carbamazepine	4-10 mcg/mL
Desipramine	150-300 ng/mL
Digoxin	0.8-2.0 ng/mL
Disopyramide	2-5 mcg/mL
Doxepin	75-200 ng/mL
Flecainide	0.2-1.0 mcg/mL
Gentamicin	Peak 6.0-8.0; trough <2.0 mcg/mL
Imipramine	150-300 ng/mL
Lidocaine	2-5 mcg/mL
Lithium	0.5-1.4 mEq/L
Nortriptyline	50-150 ng/mL
Phenobarbital	10-30 mEq/mL
Phenytoin	8-20 mcg/mL
Procainamide	4.0-8.0 mcg/mL
Quinidine	2.5-5.0 mcg/mL
Salicylate	15-25 mg/dL
Streptomycin	Peak 10-20; trough <5 mcg/mL
Theophylline	8-20 mcg/mL
Tocainide	4-10 mcg/mL
Valproic acid	50-100 mcg/mL
Vancomycin	Peak 30-40; trough <10 mcg/mL

Commonly Used Abbreviations

1/2 NS	0.45% saline solution	cc	cubic centimeter
ac	ante cibum (before meals)	CCU	coronary care unit
		cm	centimeter
ABG	arterial blood gas	CMF	cyclophosphamide, methotrexate, and fluorouracil
ac	before meals		
ACTH	adrenocorticotropic hormone	CNS	central nervous system
		CO_2	carbon dioxide
ad lib	ad libitum (as needed or desired)	COPD	chronic obstructive pulmonary disease
ADH	antidiuretic hormone	CPK	creatinine phosphokinase
AFB	acid-fast bacillus	CPK-MB	myocardial-specific CPK isoenzyme
alk phos	alkaline phosphatase		
ALT	alanine amino-transferase	CPR	cardiopulmonary resuscitation
am	morning	CSF	cerebrospinal fluid
AMA	against medical advice	CT	computerized tomography
amp	ampule	CVP	central venous pressure
AMV	assisted mandatory ventilation; assist mode ventilation	CXR	chest x-ray
		d/c	discharge; discontinue
		D5W	5% dextrose water solution; also D10W, D50W
ANA	antinuclear antibody		
ante	before	DIC	disseminated intravascular coagulation
AP	anteroposterior		
ARDS	adult respiratory distress syndrome	diff	differential count
		DKA	diabetic ketoacidosis
ASA	acetylsalicylic acid	dL	deciliter
AST	aspartate amino-transferase	DOSS	docusate sodium sulfosuccinate
bid	bis in die (twice a day)	DT's	delirium tremens
B-12	vitamin B-12 (cyanocobalamin)	ECG	electrocardiogram
		ER	emergency room
BM	bowel movement	ERCP	endoscopic retrograde cholangiopancreatography
BP	blood pressure		
BUN	blood urea nitrogen	ESR	erythrocyte sedimentation rate
c/o	complaint of		
c	cum (with)	ET	endotracheal tube
C and S	culture and sensitivity	ETOH	alcohol
C	centigrade	F	Fahrenheit
C3, C4	third and fourth complement components	Fe/TIBC	iron/total iron-binding capacity
Ca	calcium	Fe	iron
cap	capsule	FEV_1	forced expiratory volume (in one second)
CBC	complete blood count; includes hemoglobin, hematocrit, red blood cell indices, white blood cell count, and platelets	FiO2	fractional inspired oxygen
		g	gram(s)
		GC	gonococcal; gonococcus
		GFR	glomerular filtration rate

GI	gastrointestinal	LDH	lactate dehydrogenase
gm	gram	LDL	low-density lipoprotein
gt	drop	liq	liquid
gtt	drops	LLQ	left lower quadrant
h hr	hour	LP	lumbar puncture, low potency
H20	water		
HBsAG	hepatitis B surface antigen	LR	lactated Ringer's (solution)
		MB	myocardial band
HCO3	bicarbonate	MBC	minimal bacterial concentration
Hct	hematocrit		
HDL	high-density lipoprotein	mcg	microgram
Hg	mercury	mEq	milliequivalent
Hgb	hemoglobin concentration	mg	milligram
		Mg	magnesium
HIV	human immunodeficiency virus	MgSO4	Magnesium Sulfate
		MI	myocardial infarction
hr	hour	MIC	minimum inhibitory concentration
hs	hora somni (bedtime, hour of sleep)		
		mL	milliliter
IM	intramuscular	mm	millimeter
I and 0	intake and output--measurement of the patient's intake by any route (mouth, intravenous, rectum) and output by any route, including urine, vomit, diarrhea, and fluid from bleeding or drainage	MOM	Milk of Magnesia
		MRI	magnetic resonance imaging
		Na	sodium
		NaHCO3	sodium bicarbonate
		Neuro	neurologic
		NG	nasogastric
		NKA	no known allergies
		NPH	neutral protamine Hagedorn (insulin)
IU	international units	NPO	nulla per os (nothing by mouth)
ICU	intensive care unit		
IgM	immunoglobulin M	NS	normal saline solution (0.9%)
IMV	intermittent mandatory ventilation		
		NSAID	nonsteroidal anti-inflammatory drug
INH	isoniazid		
INR	International normalized ratio	O2	oxygen
		OD	right eye
IPPB	intermittent positive-pressure breathing	oint	ointment
		OS	left eye
IV	intravenous or intravenously	Osm	osmolality
		OT	occupational therapy
IVP	intravenous pyelogram; intravenous piggyback	OTC	over the counter
		OU	each eye
K, K+	potassium	oz	ounce
kcal	kilocalorie	p, post	after
KCL	potassium chloride	pc	post cibum (after meals)
KPO4	potassium phosphate	PA	posteroanterior; pulmonary artery
KUB	x-ray of abdomen (kidneys, ureters, bowels)		
		PaO2	arterial oxygen pressure
L	liter	pAO2	partial pressure of oxygen in

	alveolar gas	RL	Ringer's lactated solution (also LR)
PB	phenobarbital		
pc	after meals	ROM	range of motion
pCO2	partial pressure of carbon dioxide	rt	right
		s	sine (without)
PEEP	positive end-expiratory pressure	s/p	status post (the condition of being post)
per	by	sat	saturated
pH	hydrogen ion concentration (H+)	SBP	systolic blood pressure
		SC	subcutaneously
PID	pelvic inflammatory disease	SGOT	serum glutamic-oxaloacetic transaminase (AST)
pm	afternoon	SGPT	serum glutamic-pyruvic transaminase (ALT)
PO	orally		
PO	per os (by mouth)	SIADH	syndrome of inappropriate antidiuretic hormone
pO2	partial pressure of oxygen		
		SL	sublingually under tongue
polys	polymorphonuclear leukocytes	SLE	systemic lupus erythematosus
PPD	purified protein derivative	SMA-12	sequential multiple analysis; a panel of 12 chemistry tests performed together on a 12-channel autoanalyzer. Tests generally include Na+, K+, HCO3 , Chloride , BUN, glucose, creatinine, bilirubin, calcium, total protein, albumin, and alkaline phosphatase. Other chemistry panels include SMA-6 and SMA-20
PR	per rectum		
prn	pro re nata (as needed)		
Pro	prothrombin		
PT	physical therapy; prothrombin time		
PTCA	percutaneous transluminal coronary angioplasty		
PTT	partial thromboplastin time		
		SMX	sulfamethoxazole
PVC	premature ventricular contraction	sob	shortness of breath
		sol	solution
q	quaque (every) q6h, q2h every 6 hours; every 2 hours	SQ	under the skin
		ss	one-half
		STAT	statim (immediately)
qid	quarter in die (four times a day)	susp	suspension
		tid	ter in die (three times a day)
qAM	every morning	T4	Thyroxine level (T4)
qd	quaque die (every day)	T3RU	Triiodothyronine resin uptake
qh	every hour		
qhs	every night before bedtime	tab	tablet
		TB	tuberculosis
qid	4 times a day	Tbsp	tablespoon
qOD	every other day	Temp	temperature
qs	quantity sufficient	TIA	transient ischemic attack
R/O	rule out	tid	three times a day
RA	rheumatoid arthritis; room air; right atrial	TKO	to keep open, an infusion rate (usually 500 mL/24h)--
Resp	respiratory rate		

	just enough to keep the IV from clotting
TMP	trimethoprim
TMP-SMX	trimethoprim-sulfa-methoxazole combination
TPA	tissue plasminogen activator
TSH	thyroid-stimulating hormone
tsp	teaspoon
U	units
UA	urinalysis
ung	ointment
URI	upper respiratory infection
USP	United States Pharmacopeia
Ut Dict	as directed
UTI	urinary tract infection
VAC	vincristine, Adriamycin, and cyclophosphamide
vag	vaginal
VC	vital capacity
VDRL	Venereal Disease Research Laboratory
VF	ventricular function
V fib	ventricular fibrillation
VLDL	very low-density lipoprotein
Vol	volume
VS	vital signs
VT	ventricular tachycardia
W	water
WBC	white blood count
x	times

Index